BLUEPRINT FOR MEN'S HEALTH
A Guide to a Healthy Lifestyle
SECOND EDITION

By Armin Brott and the
Blueprint for Men's Health Advisory Board

With forewords by:
Kenneth A. Goldberg, MD
Founder, Male Health Center
and
Scott T. Williams
Vice President, Men's Health Network

MHN Men's Health Network™
www.menshealthnetwork.org

© Men's Health Network

PLEASE NOTE: Men's Health Network does not provide medical services. Rather, this information is provided to encourage you to begin a knowledgeable dialogue with your physician. Check with your health care provider about your need for specific health screenings.

ABOUT THE AUTHORS

ARMIN BROTT

Armin Brott, a spokesman for the Men's Health Network, has written about men's health for many national publications. He's also the best-selling author of seven books on fatherhood, which have helped millions of men around the world become the fathers they want to be and that their children need them to be. Visit Armin's website at www.mrdad.com.

**ADVISORY BOARD:
BLUEPRINT FOR MEN'S HEALTH**

The Advisory Board of the Blueprint for Men's Health is a group of men and women—physicians, psychologists, public health experts, safety specialists, and advocates for men's health—working together toward the common goal of improving the health, longevity, and quality of life for men and their families from all walks of life.

TABLE OF CONTENTS

1	**INTRODUCTION** III
2	**FOR WOMEN ONLY: WHY MEN'S HEALTH IS A WOMEN'S ISSUE** 1
	Identifying the Problem 1
	Recognizing Symptoms...2
	What You Can Do to Help 2
3	**YOU AND YOUR DOCTOR: PARTNERS IN HEALTH** 5
	Making a Choice..5
	Building a Relationship 6
	Preparing for Your First Visit 6
4	**PREVENTION** 7
	Steps You Can Take to Improve the Quality and Length of Your Life 7
5	**DIET AND NUTRITION**...9
	What Does a Good Diet Look Like? 9
	The New Food Pyramid 9
	Diet and Weight Loss 10
	Achieving and Maintaining a Healthy Weight 11
	What about Vitamins and Minerals? 12
	Additional Resources...12
6	**DENTAL HEALTH AND HYGIENE** 13
	Gum Disease 13
7	**EXERCISE AND FITNESS** 17
	What Kind of Exercise Should You Do? 17
	How Much Should You Exercise?...17
	Preventing Exercise-Related Injuries..19
	Treating Injuries 19
8	**SEXUAL HEALTH** 21
	Erectile Dysfunction (ED) 21
	Safe Sex and Sexually Transmitted Diseases (STDs) 22
	Birth Control/Contraception 23
	How Your Sex Life Changes as You Age 24
9	**PROSTATE HEALTH** 25
	What Is the Prostate? 25
	Prostatitis..25
	Diagnosing Prostatitis..26
	Benign Prostatic Hyperplasia (BPH) 27
	Treating BPH 27
	Prostate Cancer 29
	Risk Factors 29
	Treating Prostate Cancer...30
	Prevention 31
10	**CARDIOVASCULAR SYSTEM** 33
	Hypertension/High Blood Pressure 34
	Diagnosing and Treating High Blood Pressure......................34
	Cholesterol 34
	Coronary Heart Disease 35
	Heart Attack 36
	Angina...36
	Congestive Heart Failure...36
	Stroke...36
	Treating and Preventing Cardiovascular Disease 37

Blueprint for Men's Health: A Guide to a Healthy Lifestyle • Second Edition

TABLE OF CONTENTS

11 DIABETES **39**
   Diagnosing Diabetes 39
   Living with and Preventing Diabetes 40

12 CANCER **41**
   Risk Factors 41
   Early Detection 41
   Preventing Cancer..42

13 TESTICULAR CANCER **45**
   Risk Factors 45
   Early Detection 45

14 EMOTIONAL HEALTH AND WELL-BEING **47**
   Stress 47
   Depression..48
   Causes of Depression 49
   Treating Depression 49
   Suicide Risk 50

15 ADDICTION AND SUBSTANCE ABUSE **51**
   What is Addiction? 51
   Tobacco 51
   Alcohol 52
   Drug Abuse 53
   Hidden Addictions 54
   Treating Addictions..55

16 ACCIDENT PREVENTION AND SAFETY **57**
   Motor Vehicle Crashes 57
   Accidental Poisoning 57
   Falls 57
   Workplace Accidents 58
   Guns 58

17 FATHERHOOD..**59**
   It's Good for You..59
   It's Good for Your Children 59
   Staying Involved after Divorce or Separation 59
   Being a Good Role Model..59
   Tips to Help You Be The Kind of Dad You Want to Be 60

18 APPENDIX A: SPECIAL CONCERNS OF AFRICAN-AMERICANS, LATINOS, AND OTHER MINORITIES **61**
   You and Your Doctor 61
   Diet and Nutrition 61
   Exercise and Fitness 61
   Sexual Health 61
   Prostate Health 61
   Cardiovascular Health 62
   Diabetes..62
   Cancer 62
   Emotional Health and Wellbeing..62
   Addiction and Substance Abuse 62
   Accident Prevention and Safety 62
   Blood Disorders: Sickle Cell Anemia 62
   Facial Hair 63

19 APPENDIX B: SCREENING AND CHECKUP SCHEDULE **64**

20 APPENDIX C: RESOURCES **65**

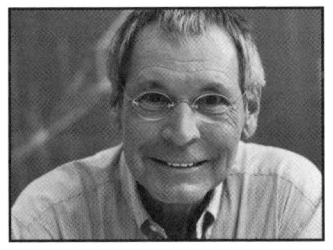

INTRODUCTION

Did you know that, on average, men are less healthy and have a shorter life expectancy than women? Part of the reason for this health gap is that we don't take care of ourselves as well as women do. Men are more likely to engage in unhealthy behavior, and less likely than women to adopt preventive health measures. We're also less likely to have health insurance, more likely to work in dangerous occupations, and often put off going to the doctor even when we really should go. As a result, men die younger—and in greater numbers—of heart disease, stroke, cancer, diabetes, and many other diseases. In 1920, women outlived men by an average of one year. Today, that difference is more than five years.

Silent Health Crisis
"There is a silent health crisis in America...it's a fact that, on average, American men live sicker and die younger than American women."
Dr. David Gremillion, Men's Health Network

More than half of premature deaths among men are preventable. But you can't prevent a problem if you don't know it exists. Throughout this book we'll discuss the main health issues that men face. Each chapter focuses on a single condition or group of related ones. We'll talk about the factors that increase your risk, show you how to recognize symptoms, and give you some practical, easy-to-implement prevention and treatment strategies.

We strongly urge you to read this book carefully—it could save your life.

In order to make the information in this book as accurate and helpful as possible, every chapter was carefully checked by a specialist with expertise in the field. However, this book is not a substitute for professional advice about medical or lifestyle issues. Seek the advice of your physician or other qualified health professional about the issues addressed in this publication.

PLEASE NOTE: Men's Health Network does not provide medical services. Rather, this information is provided to encourage you to begin a knowledgeable dialogue with your physician. Check with your health care provider about your need for specific health screenings.

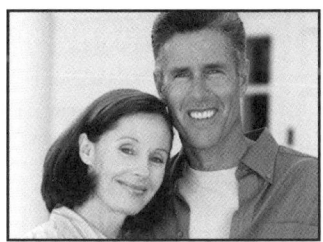

FOR WOMEN ONLY: WHY MEN'S HEALTH IS ALSO A WOMEN'S ISSUE

What does men's health have to do with you? Plenty! Men's health issues don't affect only men; they have a significant impact on everyone around them. And because women live longer than men, they see their fathers, brothers, sons, and husbands suffer or die prematurely.

More than one-half the elderly widows now living in poverty were not poor before the death of their husbands.
Meeting the Needs of Older Women: A Diverse and Growing Population, The Many Faces of Aging, U.S. Administration on Aging

---

At this point, you're probably thinking, "I already do more than my share of the laundry, the cooking, and the childcare. Can't he do anything for himself?" Of course he can. But there's a good chance that without some gentle pushing from you, he won't. So it may be up to you.

More than half of premature deaths among men are preventable. By educating yourself about potential male health problems and passing that information on to the men you love, you may be able to save a life. And by encouraging all the men in your life to realize that even the smallest symptoms can sometimes be serious and may need to be discussed with their doctors, you'll be helping them take a more active role in their own health care.

Over the next few pages, we'll summarize the potential warning signs and give you some tips on how to increase the quality and lifespan of the men in your life. But this is only a summary. We strongly encourage you to read the rest of this book carefully. Each section includes detailed information on risk factors, symptoms and prevention.

IDENTIFYING THE PROBLEM
In 1920, women outlived men by an average of one year. Today, that difference is more than five years. Why? It's because men:
- Die younger—and in greater numbers—of heart disease, stroke, cancer, diabetes, and many other diseases.
- Don't take care of themselves as well as women do.
- Are more likely to engage in unhealthy behavior.
- Don't seek medical attention when they need it.
- Are less likely than women to adopt preventive health measures.
- Are less likely to have health insurance.
- Are more likely to work in dangerous occupations.

FOR WOMEN ONLY: WHY MEN'S HEALTH IS ALSO A WOMEN'S ISSUE

RECOGNIZING SYMPTOMS

When a warning light flashes on the car dashboard, most men usually take the car to the shop. But when warning lights flash on their body, most men don't (or won't) notice. Here are a few flashing lights you should look out for:

- Changes in bowel or bladder habits. This can be an indication of prostate or bladder problems. And blood in the urine is a common indicator of kidney problems. Does he get up five times a night to go to the bathroom? That could be a symptom of an enlarged prostate, a common condition among men as they get older.
- Impotence or erectile dysfunction. Most of the time, erectile problems are caused by an underlying health problem, such as diabetes, clogged arteries, or high blood pressure. So if you want to make love and your husband says he has a headache, pay attention: it might be something far more serious.
- Persistent backaches, changes in the color of urine or stool, obvious changes in warts or moles, unusual lumps, recurrent chest pains or headaches, bleeding that won't stop, nagging cough, unexplained weight loss, and extreme fatigue can all be symptoms of other serious health problems.
- Depression. Although women may be more likely to attempt suicide, men are four times more likely to succeed. Because men are reluctant to ask for help and may try to hide their depression, you may recognize the symptoms sooner than he does. These may include acting overly anxious, having trouble sleeping, complaining of feeling sad or "empty" or helpless, engaging in unusually risky or reckless behavior, or losing interest in hobbies or other pleasurable activities (including sex).

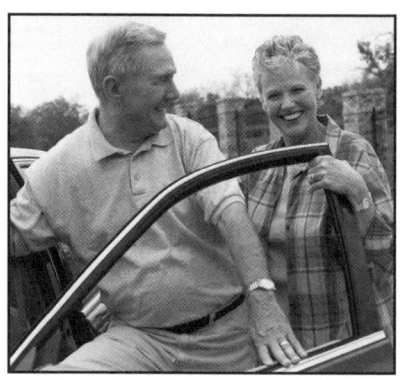

WHAT YOU CAN DO TO HELP

Know when to call in the professionals. If you identify a symptom, get your man to the doctor immediately—and don't take no for an answer. But even if he's the picture of health, one of the most important steps you can take is to get your husband (and sons) into the habit of getting regular checkups. As with most things, the results of specific exams are important, but often are not nearly as important as changes over time. In the days and weeks before the visit, help him prepare. Spend some time going over his family history (many diseases have family ties), keep track of any symptoms you're concerned about, and write down a list of questions he should ask.

Check him out. Somewhere along the line we got the idea that "self-exams" have to be done, well, by ourselves. Nothing could be further from the truth. There's no reason why he can't help you with your breast exams or you with his testicular exams. Checking each other out can serve several purposes. First, it will double the chances that his (and your) exams get done regularly and thoroughly. And

Blueprint for Men's Health: A Guide to a Healthy Lifestyle • Second Edition

FOR WOMEN ONLY: WHY MEN'S HEALTH IS ALSO A WOMEN'S ISSUE

don't forget about his back. Women get most of their skin cancers in places where they can more easily be spotted on their hands and face and below the dress line. Men get most of theirs on their backs, where they're a lot harder to see.

> *"The role of women in keeping the men in their life healthy is invaluable. While it may pain you to nag your husband about one more thing, do it anyway. If you recognize any unusual symptoms in your loved one do whatever it takes to get him the help he needs, it may save his life."*
>
> Theresa Morrow, Women Against Prostate Cancer

Prevention, prevention, prevention. Besides encouraging the men in your life to exercise, eat a high-fiber/low-fat diet, quit smoking, and do monthly self-exams, the most important step you can take is to get them into the habit of getting regular medical checkups. In Appendix B, we've included a chart of maintenance milestones that American men should follow throughout their lives to ensure good health.

We realize that many of the issues that we've covered in this book are sometimes difficult to discuss—especially for your man. But he needs to understand that he must take even the smallest symptom seriously since it could indicate a more serious—or even life-threatening—condition.

Ultimately, the goal of all this is to get your husband to take better care of himself and to get the next generation of men to start building good habits. These things sometimes take time. But even the smallest changes can bring big rewards.

If you don't have a family physician or can't afford one, look for health fairs, free or low-cost clinics, and free screening events in your area. Ask your employer, fraternal organization, or place of worship to establish a yearly health fair or screening event. Men's Health Network (MHN) can provide advice and guidance for these and other events. Call the Men's Healthline 888-MEN-2-MEN or visit the Men's Health Network web site at www.menshealthnetwork.org. MHN also maintains a list of free and low-cost clinics at www.healthclinicsonline.com.

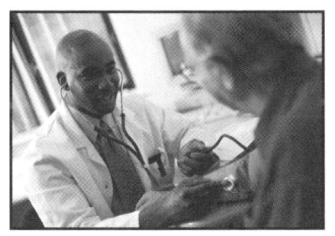

YOU AND YOUR DOCTOR: PARTNERS IN HEALTH

There's no two ways about it: we men don't take very good care of ourselves. Far too many of us don't ever see a doctor unless there's something seriously wrong or our partner or spouse makes the appointment for us. Men are half as likely to visit a doctor for a check-up as women are, and there are over 7 million American men who haven't seen a doctor in over 10 years. And even when we do go to the doctor, we often don't feel comfortable talking about our health.

Excluding pregnancy-related office visits, women make twice as many preventative care visits as men.
Utilization of Ambulatory Medical Care by Women: CDC

So why don't we take better care of ourselves? Part of the reason is the way we're brought up. As little boys, we're taught not to cry, not to complain, and not to show any signs of weakness. We ignore our aches and pains and play through our injuries. In our 20s, we think we're indestructible and see going to the doctor as a waste of time and money. In our 30s, we're too busy with our career and family to go, and by the time we're in our 40s we don't go because we're afraid of what we'll find out or we don't want to have a rectal exam (who does?).

Being tough may have some advantages. But it's also killing us. Most life-threatening illnesses, including cancer, heart disease, and diabetes, can be treated or cured if they're caught early. However, one recent study found that two-thirds of men wouldn't even go to the doctor if they were experiencing chest pain or shortness of breath—two early warning signs of a heart attack.

So here's the deal. If you can't remember the last time you had a complete physical, pick up the phone and make an appointment. (You wouldn't let 10 years go between oil changes, would you?) If something's hurting or just doesn't seem right, call. Even if you're feeling great, call anyway. The time to see your doctor isn't when you're hooked up to life support. It's now, when you're feeling healthy.

MAKING A CHOICE
Unfortunately, finding a good primary care physician isn't as easy as it should be—your insurance coverage may limit your choices, and if you don't have insurance, cost can be a big factor. But starting and maintaining a long-lasting relationship with a good doctor is critical.

So how do you find a doctor? If you have medical coverage, start by checking the list of "preferred providers" (doctors covered by the insurance). Then ask friends or co-workers for recommendations. If you're in good health, you can probably go with a general practitioner. But if you know you have a particular problem, try to choose a specialist in that area as your primary care doctor.

YOU AND YOUR DOCTOR: PARTNERS IN HEALTH

The next step is to interview a few candidates and check their references. One way to do that is by calling the American Board of Medical Specialties at 1-866-275-2267 or visit their website, www.abms.org.

If you don't have health insurance, you may be eligible for free or low-cost healthcare and prescription drug assistance. You can find information on a number of programs, as well as Medicaid and Medicare, and clinical trials at www.healthclinicsonline.com.

BUILDING A RELATIONSHIP
Actually, you're not just looking for a doctor, you're looking for a health care partner. And just like any partners, you need a partnership agreement. Here's how it works:

- It's your responsibility to give your doctor the information he or she needs to do his or her job. That means paying attention to your body and how you feel, being aware of unusual changes or aches and pains that don't go away, and finding out as much as you can about the health of other members of your family, and honestly answering questions. If you're not honest, your doctor won't be able to help you as much as if you were honest.
- It's the doctor's responsibility to use all the information you give him or her to help you stay healthy when you are, and to help you to get well when you're not.
- It's your responsibility to follow the doctor's recommendations. That means making the lifestyle changes he or she suggests, taking medication according to the directions, keeping follow-up appointments, and seeing specialists when required.

PREPARING FOR YOUR FIRST VISIT
If you're starting off a relationship with a new doctor, here are some suggestions that will help you make the best use of your first appointment:

- Try to schedule your first appointment at a time when you're not sick. This will give the doctor a baseline, allowing a comparison of your symptoms when you're ill to what is known about you when you're well.
- Write down all the questions, worries, or concerns you have—even the private or embarrassing ones about sex or drug use. What you tell your doctor is completely confidential (unless you're doing something to endanger another person).
- Write down your family's medical history, including illnesses, diseases, chronic conditions, premature deaths, and so on. Our "Time Out for Men's Health" self-assessment can help you collect all that information in one place. It's available for free at www.healthselfassessment.com. Complete this self assessment and take it with you when you go to the doctor.
- Bring in all the medications you're taking, as well as vitamins, supplements and herbs.
- Make a list of all your symptoms, allergies, or reactions to medications.
- Be honest about smoking, drinking, drug use, sexual history, diet and exercise.
- Write down the doctor's suggestions, advice, and answers to your questions.
- Most doctors will be thrilled to have a patient who is truly participating in his health care. If your doctor doesn't listen to you, find another one.

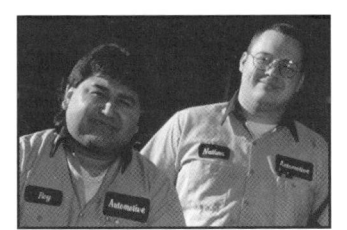

PREVENTION

Men die younger than women from the top causes of death. As a result, the average woman outlives the average man by over five years. But it doesn't have to be this way. More than half of these premature deaths are preventable, along with about 60 percent of chronic diseases, and most injuries and accidents. By taking charge of your own preventative care, you can protect your health.

Among men, more than one-half of premature deaths are preventable.

STEPS YOU CAN TAKE TO IMPROVE THE QUALITY AND LENGTH OF YOUR LIFE

Below is a summary of important steps you can take to improve the quality—and length—of your life. We'll discuss these steps in more detail throughout this book.

- Eat a varied diet, rich in fruits, vegetables, whole grains, and low-fat foods.
- Be especially careful to limit cholesterol intake and avoid saturated fats.
- Moderate exercise for 30 minutes five times a week, or vigorous exercise for 20 minutes three times a week.
- Protect yourself from the sun.
- Maintain a healthy weight.
- Drink at least eight 8-ounce glasses of water per day.
- Limit alcohol to two drinks per day.
- Don't smoke, and minimize your exposure to second-hand smoke.
- See your doctor regularly.
- Know your family history and discuss it with your doctor.
- If you are over 40, get a baseline PSA (prostate specific antigen) test and monitor this periodically with your doctor.
- Practice safe sex.
- Wear a seatbelt whenever you're in the car, and a helmet when on a motorcycle or bicycle.
- Manage your stress.
- Get help if you need it.

As important as it is for you to take charge of your own health and wellness, you can't do it all. Getting regular checkups and age-appropriate screenings is a proven way to improve health and reduce premature death and disability.

At the back of this book you'll find a schedule of the most common screenings you should have and how often you should have them. Remember, if you're a member of a high-risk group or have a family history of disease, talk to your health care provider about the benefits of earlier screenings.

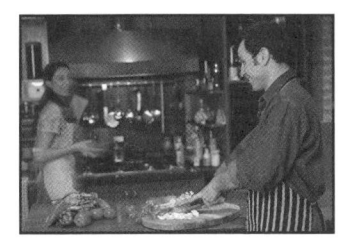

DIET AND NUTRITION

There's a lot of truth to the old expression that "You are what you eat."

Over 60 percent of adult American men are overweight.

Everything that you eat or drink has an effect on your health and well being, which is why it's so important to make eating a balanced, nutritious diet a priority in your life. Unfortunately, too many of us don't do that. We tend to eat portions that are too large, and our diets include too much fat, sugar and salt.

WHAT DOES A GOOD DIET LOOK LIKE?

Take U.S. Department of Agriculture's Food Pyramid provides guidance.

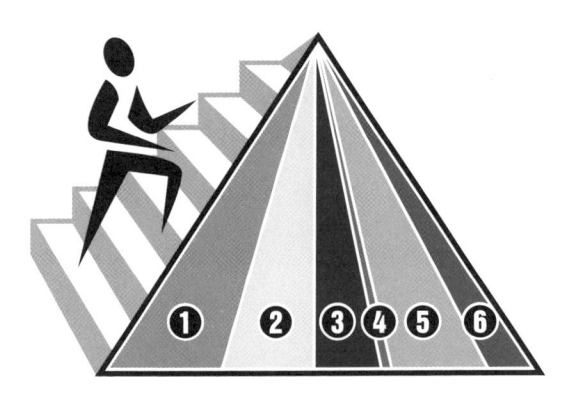

MyPyramid.gov
Steps to a Healthier You

The Food Pyramid is divided into six stripes, each of the six stripes represents a different type of food, and the little guy going up the stairs is a reminder that a healthy diet and plenty of exercise are both important in maintaining health. Let's take a closer look at each of the 6 food categories:

① GRAINS: Eat at least three ounces of grains—this includes cereals, crackers, rice, or pasta every day, half of which are made of whole grains. Not sure how much grain is an ounce? It's a slice of bread, 1 cup of ready-to-eat cereal, or 1/2 cup of cooked rice, pasta, or cereal. Grains—especially whole grains—are rich in fiber, reduce the risk of heart disease and can help you maintain a healthy weight.

DIET AND NUTRITION

② **VEGETABLES:** Eat about 2 to 3 cups of vegetables per day. It doesn't matter whether your veggies are fresh, frozen, canned, cooked or dried. The important thing is to get a good mix of dark green (such as spinach, mustard greens, and broccoli), orange (such as carrots, pumpkin, and yams), starchy (like corn and potatoes), beans and peas (includes tofu, black beans, kidney beans), and any others, such as tomatoes, bell peppers, and mushrooms. Eating a variety of vegetables every day may reduce the risk of stroke, heart attack, and diabetes, and may protect you against colorectal and other cancers.

③ **FRUIT:** Eat 2 cups of fruit every day. Any fruit or 100 percent juice counts. And you can use fresh, canned, cut or frozen. Count 1/2 cup of dried fruit as a whole cup, and limit yourself to one cup of fruit juice per day. As with vegetables, eating a variety of fruits every day may reduce the risk of stroke, heart attack, and diabetes, and may protect you against colorectal and other cancers.

④ **FATS AND OILS:** Seven teaspoons of oil per day for men 19-30; 6 teaspoons for men 31 and older. This includes any kind of liquid oil, as well as nuts, olives, avocados, mayonnaise and many salad dressings. The yellow stripe is very narrow to remind you that you should be especially careful with this group. Four large olives is 1 teaspoon, and a small handful of nuts is three. Limit solid fats such as shortening, lard, butter, and margarine. When looking at labels, try to stick with polyunsaturated and monounsaturated fats, and avoid saturated and trans fats, since they increase your risk of heart disease.

⑤ **DAIRY:** Consume three cups of dairy products per day. Milk and yogurt are measured in cups, 1 - 2 ounces of cheese counts as a cup. Limit dairy products that have little or no calcium, such as cream cheese and butter, and choose fat-free or low-fat options whenever possible. If you're lactose intolerant (meaning you have a tough time digesting any milk products), lactose-free options are available. Getting plenty of milk products helps build and strengthen healthy bones. This is important throughout your life, but especially during adolescence.

⑥ **MEAT, POULTRY, FISH:** Eat 5 to 6 ounces of lean meat, poultry, fish, dry beans, eggs or nuts every day—a little more if you exercise more than 30 minutes. Each ounce of meat, poultry and fish counts as one ounce. But 1/2 ounce of seeds or nuts, 1 tablespoon of peanut butter, 1 egg, or 1/4 cup of cooked beans is the equivalent of an ounce. Broil, grill, or bake meats and poultry instead of frying. The foods in this group are important sources of protein, which help build muscles, bones, skin and blood. They are also an excellent source of vitamins B and E, and other nutrients, including iron, zinc, magnesium, which protect your body's cells, carry oxygen to your blood, and strengthen your immune system.

DIET AND WEIGHT LOSS

Over 60 percent of American men are overweight or obese. Mexican-American men are the most likely to be overweight, followed by white men and African-American men. Being overweight causes more than 300,000 premature deaths every year, increases the risk of developing diabetes, heart disease, stroke and cancer, and can worsen other conditions such as depression.

Americans spend over $30 billion on diet programs, and it sometimes seems that you can't open up a magazine or turn on the television without seeing an ad for a new miracle diet or program or pill or gadget that will supposedly help you "lose those extra pounds and keep them off." Unfortunately, most of these offers are scams. They don't work, they're sometimes dangerous, and the only thing you'll lose is money.

Ignore any weight-loss program that claims you can eat all you want and still get thin, or that you'll lose weight while you sleep, or that it's "a new discovery," "miraculous," "exclusive," "secret," "magical," "easy," or anything that sounds too good to be true.

The only truly effective way to lose weight permanently is to reduce the number of calories you eat and get more exercise. And you'll have to be patient: it'll take you about the same amount of time to lose the weight as it did to gain it, which is about one or two pounds per week. Losing weight faster than that isn't healthy, and won't last.

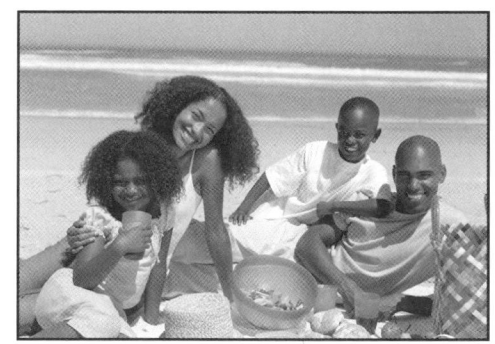

One pound of fat is about 3,500 calories. So if every day you can cut 250 calories out of your diet (the equivalent of one candy bar) and burn another 250 (by doing as little as 20 to 30 minutes of walking), you'll lose a pound a week. Keep that up for six months and you'll have lost 25 pounds!

Before starting any weight loss program, check with your doctor.

YOUR DIET AND YOUR BONES
When it comes to your bones, the old expression "you are what you eat" couldn't be more true. Not getting enough calcium increases your risk of developing osteoporosis, a disease that reduces bone mass, which in turn increases your risk of bone fracture. For most men, about 1,500 milligrams per day is a good goal. And you can get most of that by eating calcium rich foods such as milk (including soy), cheese, fish, and green vegetables such as broccoli and kale. You can also get calcium-fortified cereals and juices. The amount of calcium you need depends on your age, overall health, and other factors, so be sure to check with your healthcare provider before making big changes to your diet or taking calcium supplements.

ACHIEVING AND MAINTAINING A HEALTHY WEIGHT
Maintaining a healthy weight doesn't require a lot of effort. Below you'll find a number of ways that will help. The more you can follow, the easier it will be:

- Follow the guidelines in the new Food Pyramid, and limit your fat intake to no more than 30 percent of the calories you eat every day. Choose non-fat or low-fat options whenever possible. Have baked potatoes instead of

DIET AND NUTRITION

French fries, get your salad dressing on the side and don't use all of it, and skip the cheese on your burger.
- Eat slowly, pay attention to how you feel, don't have seconds unless you're really hungry, and stop when you're full. Despite what your mother may have said, you do not always need to finish everything on your plate.
- Eat smaller portions.
- Don't skip breakfast. People who eat a healthy breakfast tend to eat less during the day, have lower cholesterol (see page 34), and are able to concentrate better at work and at home.
- Eat out less often. Home-cooked meals tend to be lower in calories and fat than restaurant-cooked foods.
- Drink less alcohol. Several research studies show that moderate alcohol consumption may have some health benefits. "Moderate" means no more than two drinks per day. If controlling your drinking is a problem for you, avoid alcohol entirely.
- Limit caffeine. One or two cups a day won't hurt you, but more than that can cause dehydration, insomnia, anxiety and heart palpitations (irregular heart beat).
- Get into the habit of reading the ingredients panel on food packages, and avoid high-calorie, high-fat, high-sodium snack foods or fast foods.
- Avoid any food that contains hydrogenated or partially hydrogenated oils. These are called "trans fat" and are extremely unhealthy.
- Drink at least eight glasses of water every day.
- Eat more fresh fruits and vegetables.

WHAT ABOUT VITAMINS AND MINERALS?

Just as with diets, there's a lot of inaccurate information out there about vitamins and nutritional supplements. While there's no question that getting enough vitamins and minerals is essential, you probably don't need to take any supplements if you're eating a healthy, balanced diet.

However, if any of the following are true, you may need vitamin and/or mineral supplements:

- You regularly eat less than 1,200 calories per day.
- You regularly skip meals.
- You take medication that interferes with your body's ability to absorb vitamins and minerals.
- You are lactose intolerant (meaning you can't digest milk or dairy products) and aren't getting enough calcium.
- If you chose to take vitamins, take only the recommended daily allowance (it's printed on the package). Taking higher does for long periods of time can be harmful. And be sure to check with your doctor before taking any nutritional supplements.

ADDITIONAL RESOURCES

- Check with your doctor before going on any diet or taking any vitamins or supplements.
- More detailed nutritional information is available online at www.mypyramid.gov.

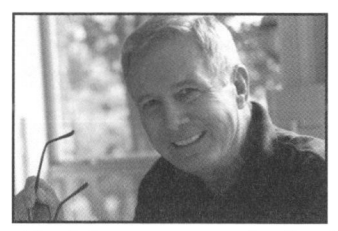

DENTAL HEALTH AND HYGIENE

From the time you were a little boy, you've been hearing about how important it is to brush your teeth and floss every day. But caring for your teeth and gums does more than improve your smile and your breath. In fact, good dental hygiene may actually reduce your risk of ulcers, pneumonia, digestive problems, heart disease, stroke and diabetes.

A healthy mouth doesn't just happen by itself—you need to take on an active role by making dental hygiene a part of your everyday routine. By working with your dentist and following the suggestions in this chapter, you'll improve your chances of keeping your teeth—and your health—for a lifetime.

WHAT'S REALLY GOING ON IN YOUR MOUTH?
Although you can't see them, there are literally millions of bacteria in your mouth. Some are harmless and help break down the food you eat so it can be more easily digested. Other bacteria are quite harmful. They clump together to create plaque, a sticky, acidic substance that builds up on the teeth.

Having plaque on your teeth is perfectly normal—everyone does—and if it's regularly removed (by brushing and flossing every day), plaque is harmless. But if it's not removed, plaque begins eating away and decaying your teeth and will ultimately cause cavities and gum disease. Over time, the bones and tissue that hold your teeth can be destroyed. Your teeth may become loose and/or fall out.

GUM DISEASE
In fact, good dental hygiene may actually reduce your risk of ulcers, pneumonia, digestive problems, heart disease, stroke and diabetes . Approximately 75 percent of adults over 35 will have some form of gum disease at some point in their life. Here are some of the risk factors:

- Being male. Men are more likely to suffer from gum disease than women.
- Being African-American. Black men are more likely than white men to develop gum disease.
- Being poor or uninsured. People at the lowest socio-economic levels tend to have the most severe gum disease. This is largely because they don't have access to (or can't afford) regular dental care.
- Age. As we get older, our gums gradually recede, exposing the roots of the teeth to plaque. We also produce less saliva, which plays an important role in rinsing plaque out of the mouth.
- Genetics. If your parents lost teeth to gum disease, you are at greater risk.
- Not brushing and flossing regularly.
- Poor diet.
- Clenching, grinding teeth.
- Smoking.

DENTAL HEALTH AND HYGIENE

Symptoms of Gum Disease:
In the early stages, gum disease is painless and you might not even notice if you have it. But if you notice any of the following symptoms, you should see a dentist as soon as you can.

- Red, swollen, tender gums.
- Gums that bleed when you brush or floss.
- Gums that have receded (pulled away) from the teeth.
- Persistent bad breath or bad taste in the mouth.
- Pockets of pus around teeth or gums.
- Loose teeth, changes in the way your teeth fit together when you bite.
- Pain when chewing or difficulty chewing certain kinds of foods (usually crunchy foods).

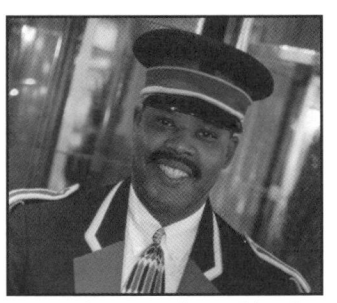

PREVENTION AND TREATMENT:
Fortunately, most cavities can be prevented and early gum disease can almost always be reversed—but you'll have to make a commitment to taking better care of your teeth. Here are some important steps to take:

- Have your teeth checked and cleaned at least twice a year—more often if your dentist suggests it.
- Brush at least twice a day with fluoride toothpaste—if possible after every meal. Use a soft bristled brush. Be sure to clean the inside surfaces of the teeth (the side closest to your tongue) as well as the outside surfaces. Replace your brush every three months or whenever the bristles fray.
- Floss every day. Plaque usually builds up along the gumline (where the teeth and gums meet) and in-between the teeth. Your toothbrush can take care of the gumline, but it can't get to the spaces between the teeth. Dental floss can. If you aren't sure how to floss, your dentist or hygienist can show you.
- Brush your tongue or use a scraper to remove the bacteria that gathers towards the back of your tongue.
- Eat crunchy foods like apples and carrots. They actually help reduce plaque buildup on the surfaces of the teeth and may even help reduce coffee stains.
- Avoid sugary snacks and soft drinks between meals. These foods quickly convert to plaque. If you crave something sweet, try a piece of fruit instead.
- Drink lots of water. Saliva helps reduce plaque by washing it away. But age and some medications may make your mouth dry and more susceptible to plaque buildup, tooth decay and gum disease. Chewing sugarless gum is one way to stimulate saliva.
- Don't smoke or chew tobacco. Besides staining your teeth, it can cause bad breath and lead to oral cancer.
- Avoid chewing hard candies or anything else that might damage your teeth.

- Protect yourself. In many sports there's a risk of mouth injuries (from pucks, balls, racquets and elbows). You can reduce the chance of doing long-term damage to your teeth by always wearing a mouth guard.
- If you have dentures, most of the suggestions above apply to dentures as well as your natural teeth.

OTHER POSSIBLE DENTAL PROBLEMS:
- Sensitivity to hot or cold. When gums recede, they expose some of the root of the tooth, which can be extremely sensitive to temperature changes.
- Bad breath (also called halitosis). Bad breath can be caused by smoking, eating spicy or smelly foods, or poor brushing. However, if you have bad breath that won't go away no matter how much you brush your teeth or how much mouthwash you use, you may have a serious dental or medical problem. See your dentist right away.

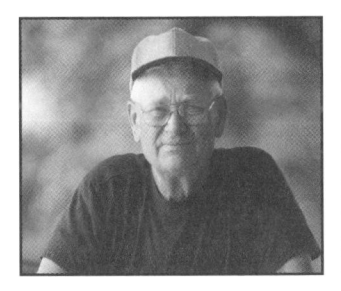

EXERCISE AND FITNESS

Regular physical activity is the closest thing there is to a miracle drug.

Regular physical activity, whether it's walking up a few flights of stairs or running a marathon, is the closest thing that exists to a miracle drug. Research has shown that exercise:

- Helps prevent heart disease and stroke.
- Lowers blood pressure.
- Helps control diabetes.
- Lowers stress levels.
- Reduces symptoms of anxiety and depression and improves mood.
- Prevents obesity.
- Reduces the risk of developing certain cancers, including colon cancer.
- Improves brain function.
- Helps fight off some of the most common signs of aging, such as arthritis, loss of bone density (called osteoporosis) and memory loss.

Despite all these benefits, over half of Americans get less exercise than they should, and a quarter get none at all. African-American and Hispanic-American men are somewhat less likely to exercise than white men.

WHAT KIND OF EXERCISE SHOULD YOU DO?
There are two basic kinds of exercise:

- **Aerobic exercise** involves increasing your heart rate and breathing and keeping them at higher levels for an extended period. Aerobic exercise strengthens the heart and burns fat. Examples include fast walking, running, hiking, bike riding, swimming, skiing, basketball, karate, even jumping rope.
- **Anaerobic exercise** involves short periods of intense exercise followed by a period of rest. Anaerobic builds muscle and strengthens bones. Examples include weight lifting and sprinting.

Both kinds of exercise are important and you should try to get some of both every day.

HOW MUCH SHOULD YOU EXERCISE?
Before starting any exercise program, talk it over with your doctor for guidance.

If you haven't been very active until now, start off easy—you may only be able to do five minutes per day. But gradually increase your time until you're up to 20 minutes or more per day. Your goal is to increase your heart rate and breathing. You want to feel slightly out of breath, but not so out of breath that you can't carry on a conversation.

EXERCISE AND FITNESS

Ideally, you should try to get 30 to 60 minutes of exercise on most days (the more the better, but try for at least three to five). That may seem like a lot, especially if you haven't been exercising regularly. But the good news is that you don't have to do it all at one time. Instead, you can spread it out over the course of your day. Research has shown that even simply walking quickly for as little as 30 minutes per day decreases your risk of having a heart attack, stroke and diabetes.

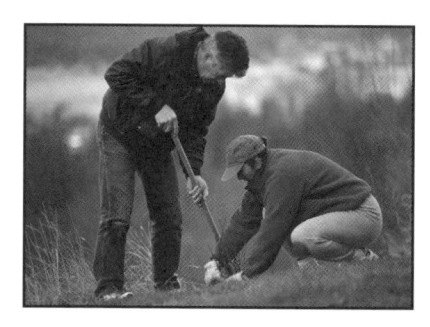

Any kind of activity—even mowing the lawn, washing your car, or wrestling with your children—is better than none. But you won't benefit very much from doing exercise unless you do it more than two times per week or more than 10 minutes per day. And if you're interested in losing weight, you'll need to get at least 30 minutes of continuous aerobic exercise a minimum of five days per week.

The best way to ensure that you're getting the most out of each workout is to get your heart rate into the target zone and keep it there for 30 minutes. Calculating your target rate is a two-step process.

- Find your maximum heart rate. To do that, simply subtract your age from 220. So if you're 44 years old, your maximum heart rate is 176.
- Your target zone is 50 to 80 percent of your maximum heart rate. So if your max rate is 176, your target zone is 88 to 141 beats per minute.

Finding an activity or two that you enjoy is the key to making exercise a lifelong habit. Most people don't do this, though, and that's why more than half of those who start an exercise program don't stick with it for more than six months. Fortunately, there are dozens of easy ways to increase the amount of exercise you get every day. Here are just a few examples:

- Take the stairs instead of the elevator or escalator whenever you can.
- When you go out shopping, park your car as far away as you can from where you're going. If you take public transportation, get off a few stops early and walk the rest of the way.
- Do some sit-ups, pushups, squats, or jumping jacks, or use a ski-machine or treadmill while you're watching television.
- Participate in a Walk-A-Thon.
- Carry your own groceries instead of letting a clerk do it for you.
- Use a manual lawn-mower instead of a power model.
- Skip that mid-morning cup of coffee and go for a walk around the office instead.
- Join a group or find a workout partner.
- Take a dance class with your partner.

EXERCISE AND FITNESS

"All it takes is 30 minutes of movement or activity a day, whether it be structured or unstructured exercise and you're on your way to a healthier and stronger you."
Karla Y. Ortiz, CHES, Men's Health Network

PREVENTING EXERCISE-RELATED INJURIES
One of the biggest reasons why people give up on their exercise programs is that they try to do too much too quickly, and they injure themselves in the process. Following these tips will help you prevent injuries:

- Get the right equipment. If you're running or walking, for example, good shoes are essential for protecting your knees and other joints. Wear a helmet, groin cup, goggles, or whatever is necessary to minimize injury.
- Warm up for five to 10 minutes before you start your workout. This can be anything from a brisk walk and a few jumping jacks to running a mile at a slow pace. After you've warmed up, do some stretching. Warm muscles are less likely to get strained or injured.
- Cool down after your workout. Muscles often tighten up after exercise, so doing some light stretching will keep you limber and reduce the chance of injury.
- Whenever you lift anything, bend your knees and use your legs, not your back.
- Drink plenty of water before, during, and after your workouts.
- Vary your routine. Boredom can make you pay less attention to safety.
- Listen to your body. Forget "no pain, no gain." If you feel pain, or experience dizziness, tightening in your chest, or anything else that doesn't seem right, stop what you're doing immediately.
- Set reasonable, achievable goals. If you haven't exercised in a few years, don't expect to get out there and perform as well as you did in high school. Ease into it, and be patient with yourself.

TREATING INJURIES
Of course, despite your best efforts, injuries sometimes happen. So if you strain, pull or irritate something, remember RICE:

- **REST.** Stop exercising. Don't "play through" your injuries.
- **ICE.** Put an ice pack on the injured area for 20 minutes out of each hour for the first day or two after the injury.
- **COMPRESSION.** Wrap the injured area in an Ace bandage.
- **ELEVATION.** Try to keep the injured area higher than your heart so that blood won't pool there.

In addition, you can take over-the-counter painkillers such as aspirin and ibuprofen to reduce the swelling.

After 24 to 48 hours of following the RICE routine, gently stretch the injured area. Stop before it becomes painful.

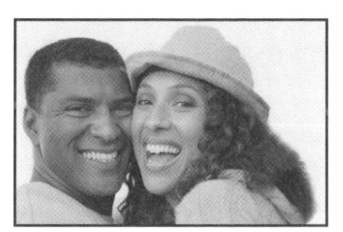

SEXUAL HEALTH

For up to 30 million American men, erectile dysfunction is an ongoing problem.

Generally speaking, your sex life is a reflection of your overall health—the healthier you are, the better it will be. But good overall health isn't a guarantee of a good sex life. In this chapter we'll discuss men's most common sexual problems and how to overcome them.

ERECTILE DYSFUNCTION (ED)

Sometimes called impotence, ED means that you can't regularly get or keep an erection long enough to satisfy your sexual needs or those of your partner. All men—whether they admit it or not—have an occasional erection problem. But for as many as 30 million American men—10 percent of all men, up to 15-25 percent of men over 65, ED is an ongoing problem. It can start at any age in adult men and can develop slowly over time or suddenly.

There are a lot of myths out there about ED. Some people insist that "it's all in your head." Others say that "it's what happens when you get older." The truth is that about 70 percent of the time, ED is the result of a physical problem that can almost always be treated. Heart disease, high blood pressure, diabetes, smoking, alcoholism, back injuries, testosterone deficiency, prostate problems including surgery, and over 200 prescription drugs can all contribute to or cause ED.

Even though physical problems are behind most ED, psychological factors including depression and performance anxiety still play a role. Men who suffer from ED often feel inadequate and less sure of themselves. That can make them anxious, tense, angry or worried that they can't satisfy their partners. Those feelings only make the ED worse. And a "mild" case of ED due to physical factors will usually be made worse by performance anxiety.

If you're experiencing ED, do yourself and your partner a favor and schedule a visit to your doctor right now. Chances are, he'll be able to get to the bottom of your ED problem in just one or two visits. He'll ask you a lot of questions about your health habits, diet, prescription drugs and under what circumstances the ED happens. He may also order tests of your blood, urine, heart function and hormone levels.

Treating ED

In many cases, taking steps to improve your overall health will help reduce or even eliminate ED. This means:

- Eat a low-fat, low-sodium, low-cholesterol diet.
- Quit smoking. Chemicals in cigarette smoke can narrow blood vessels, making it harder to maintain an erection.
- Drink less alcohol. Alcohol slows your body's reaction times.

SEXUAL HEALTH

- Get more exercise. Exercise builds muscle, improves blood flow, and helps get the cholesterol out of your blood. It also improves your mood, which will make you feel better about yourself.
- Cut back on coffee.
- Use it or lose it. The more erections you get, the easier it is to get them. Sexual activity, including masturbation, increases blood flow and oxygen to the penis.

If these lifestyle changes aren't successful, your doctor may prescribe one or more drugs to treat ED. These include sildenafil citrate (Viagra), tadalafil (Cialis), and vardenafil Hcl (Levitra). Each has advantages, disadvantages, and potential side effects that your doctor will explain. Alternatively, your doctor could prescribe injections, vacuum devices or one of a number of surgical options.

SAFE SEX AND SEXUALLY TRANSMITTED DISEASES (STDs)

Sexually transmitted diseases (STDs) are infections that are spread through sexual contact, including vaginal intercourse, oral sex, anal sex, and sometimes even kissing. The more sexual partners you have, the greater your risk of getting an STD.

STDs are widespread—19 million new cases are diagnosed every year—and there are over 20 different varieties. STDs often have no symptoms early on, which means they can be passed on to a partner without knowing it.

Below you'll find information on the most common STDs, their symptoms, and how to prevent them. If you suspect that you have one, see your doctor immediately and tell your partner so she or he can get checked as well.

- **Chlamydia** is the most common STD in the US. Thirty percent of women who get it and are not treated become sterile (are unable to have children), and it can also cause sterility in men. About three-quarters of infected women and about half of infected men have no symptoms. If symptoms do occur, they usually appear within one to three weeks after exposure. Symptoms are a thin, clear discharge of fluid from the penis and a burning feeling in the penis or scrotum. Chlamydia is easily diagnosed with a urine test and treatments are widely available.
- **Gonorrhea** is one of the most common infectious diseases in the world. It's also one of the easiest to cure—as long as it's caught early. Untreated, it can cause infertility, and it can spread to other parts of the body. Symptoms can appear two to 30 days after the infection, and include a burning feeling when urinating and a yellowish or greenish discharge from the penis. If any of that fluid gets into an eye, it can cause blindness. Gonorrhea is treated with antibiotics.
- **Syphilis** is a serious bacterial infection. Symptoms begin with bumps or sores on the penis, mouth, or anus that last anywhere from one to five weeks. These sores sometimes leak fluid that is highly contagious. Fever, rash, and flu-like symptoms follow. Caught early, syphilis can be treated with antibiotics. But untreated, it can damage the brain, heart and spinal cord—and even cause death.
- **Herpes** is caused by a virus. Symptoms begin to appear within a week of infection. They start with tingling and itching, followed by small, painful

blisters that can appear on the penis, mouth, anus, butt or thighs. Herpes can be confirmed only by examining a sample taken from the sores under a microscope. There is no cure for herpes and outbreaks can happen several times or more per year. It can be controlled by taking special anti-viral medication. Unfortunately, herpes can be contagious even when there are no sores present, so if you're diagnosed, protect your partner from infection by wearing a condom.
- **Genital warts** are exactly what they sound like—growths or bumps on the penis, but may also appear in other areas, like the anus or the thigh. Caused by a viral infection, genital warts spread quickly. The first symptoms are itching and irritation, which start within a month after infection. The warts appear soon afterwards. They can be treated with prescription medication or surgically removed. Unfortunately, genital warts can lead to cancer in women.
- **Acquired Immunodeficiency Syndrome (AIDS)** develops from exposure to the HIV virus, which lives in bodily fluids such as semen, breast milk, vaginal secretions, blood, saliva, and even tears. Speak to your health care provider about how the HIV virus can be transmitted. AIDS is a fatal disease. However, identified early and aggressively treated, the HIV virus can sometimes be kept from developing into AIDS. The HIV virus is typically treated with combination drug therapy.

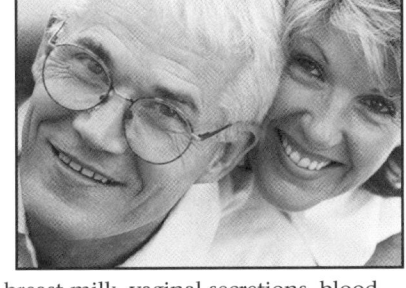

Abstinence (avoiding all sexual contact, including oral sex), is the only way to avoid STDs. However, that isn't a practical solution for many people. So if you're sexually active, you must protect yourself and your partners. Wearing a latex condom can reduce or eliminate the possibility of being infected with, or spreading, an STD. Do not use petroleum-based lubricants (like Vaseline) which can weaken the durability of a latex condom and thereby increase your risk of infection.

BIRTH CONTROL/CONTRACEPTION
When it comes to having sex, STDs aren't the only things you have to protect yourself from. You and your partner are equally responsible for doing what's necessary to prevent an unplanned pregnancy. Fortunately, there are a number of safe and reliable methods. Here are a few of the most common:

- **The pill.** When taken properly by your partner, birth control pills are nearly 100 percent effective.
- **Implants and injections.** If a woman wants to avoid the inconvenience of taking pills every day, she can have certain hormones implanted under her skin that are effective for as long as five years. Pregnancy-preventing hormones can also be injected, but they are effective for only three months at a time.
- **Condoms.** Worn properly and used with a contraceptive foam or jelly, condoms can prevent pregnancy up to 99 percent of the time. To prevent

SEXUAL HEALTH

pregnancy, you need to wear a condom every time you have sex. And never use it more than once.
- **Vasectomy.** This is a surgical procedure that involves disconnecting the tubes that carry sperm from the testicles to the penis. It's usually done in the doctor's office and is generally quick and painless. A vasectomy is virtually 100 percent effective in preventing pregnancy, but it won't protect you against STDs. If you decide you want to have children later, it's possible to reconnect the tubes, but there's less than a 50-50 chance of success.
- **Patches, pills, injections, and implants for men.** These options aren't available yet, but they will be in the near future.

Remember, protecting yourself from unwanted pregnancy is as much your responsibility as it is your partner's. So make sure you and your partner talk about birth control before you start getting undressed. If you wait longer than that, it's going to be hard to stop.

"There's no fighting the fact that your sex life will change as you age... but that change doesn't necessarily have to be bad. The key is communication. If there's something wrong, talk to a doctor, but don't forget to talk to your partner as well. Open communication about how you're feeling may lead to a different sex life. You and your partner may start focusing more on other intimate behaviors rather than just sex, but that may be an enjoyable thing for both of you!"

Susan Milstein, EdD, CHES, CSE

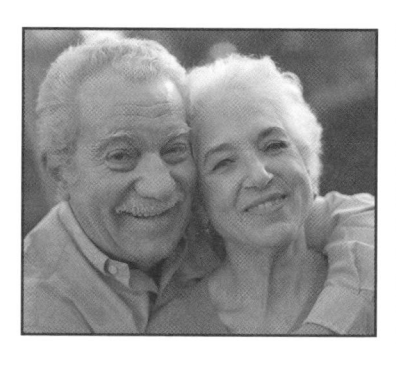

HOW YOUR SEX LIFE CHANGES AS YOU AGE

There's no question that your sex life will change as you get older. You probably won't respond to sexual stimulation as quickly as you did when you were younger. You may lose your erection after sex sooner and it may take longer for you to get another erection. But none of this means that you can't have an active sex life. The key is to keep it going. Without regular workouts, your sexual muscles will get weaker.

As men, having a positive self-image is a very important part of our sex life. But the two are connected in a kind of loop: the more attractive and desirable we feel, the better we'll perform. At the same time, the better we perform sexually, the more attractive and desirable we feel. For this reason, it's especially important to talk with your doctor about any sexual problems. As we discussed above, most are treatable.

Blueprint for Men's Health: A Guide to a Healthy Lifestyle • Second Edition

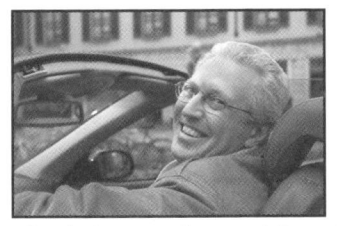

PROSTATE HEALTH

> *BPH (prostate enlargement) is the most frequent prostate condition in men over 50.*

If you don't know what your prostate is or what it does, you're certainly not alone. Most men don't. But you really should. Over 30 million men suffer from prostate conditions that negatively affect their quality of life. And every year over 230,000 men will be diagnosed with prostate cancer and about 30,000 will die of it.

WHAT IS THE PROSTATE?

Technically, the prostate is a part of your sex organs, producing fluid that contributes to the production of sperm. It's a small gland, about the size of a walnut, that surrounds your urethra, a tube that takes urine from the bladder to the penis. The urethra also carries semen during ejaculation. The prostate gland grows quite a lot during puberty and then doesn't change much until about age 40, when it slowly begins growing again and, in many men, continues to grow as they age. Half of men aren't bothered by their growing prostate. But the others will develop one of three prostate diseases, or may have more than one.

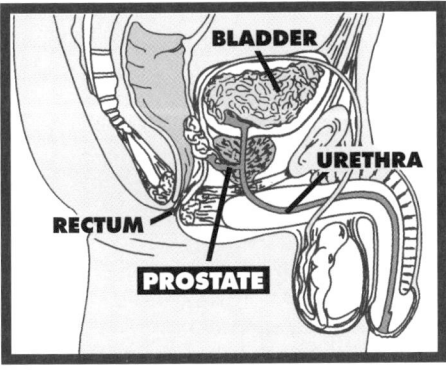

PROSTATITIS

Prostatitis is an inflammation of the prostate that may be caused by an infection. It's the most common prostate problem for men under 50—so common that about half of adult men will be treated for it during their lifetime.

There are three major types of prostatitis:

- Bacterial prostatitis
- Nonbacterial prostatitis
- Prostatodynia

Bacterial prostatitis. There are actually two types of bacterial prostatitis: acute (meaning it develops suddenly) and chronic (meaning it develops slowly over several years). Both types can be treated with antibiotics. Each type affects about 1 in 10 men with prostatitis. Symptoms of acute bacterial prostatitis are often severe, and therefore are usually quickly diagnosed. These symptoms include:

- Fever
- Chills
- Aching muscles
- Fatigue
- Pain in lower back
- Frequent and/or painful urination

Chronic bacterial prostatitis may involve few symptoms other than those of a recurring urinary tract infection (frequent and painful urination), and the condition keeps returning even after the initial infection has been treated and symptoms have disappeared.

Nonbacterial prostatitis occurs in about 6 out of 10 men with prostatitis. Although the causes are unknown, the inflammation may be related to organisms other than bacteria, like a reaction to the urine or substances in the urine. For example, men with a history of allergies and asthma sometimes develop nonbacterial prostatitis. However, doctors cannot be sure exactly how these conditions are related. Doctors know that nonbacterial prostatitis is not found in men with recurrent bladder infections. Symptoms include:

- Occasional discomfort in the testicles, urethra, lower abdomen, and back.
- Discharge from the urethra, especially during the first bowel movement of the day.
- Blood or urine in ejaculate.
- Low sperm count.
- Sexual difficulties.
- Frequent urination.

Prostatodynia (pain in the area of the prostate gland) occurs in about 3 out of 10 men with prostate irritation. Unfortunately, tests used to diagnose infection and other problems affecting the prostate gland are not useful in detecting the cause of this pain. In some instances, the pain may be caused by a muscle spasm (an involuntary sudden movement or contraction) in the bladder or the urethra. Usually, though, the cause of prostatodynia is unknown. Symptoms include pain and discomfort in the prostate gland, testicles, penis, and urethra, and may include difficulty urinating.

Certain activities increase your risk of developing prostatitis. These include:

- Having had a recent bladder infection.
- Having benign prostatic hyperplasia (BPH, see next section).
- Having gonorrhea, chlamydia or another sexually transmitted disease.
- Having frequent, unprotected sex or unprotected sex with multiple partners.
- Excessive alcohol consumption.
- Eating a lot of spicy, marinated foods.
- Injury to the lower pelvis (often as a result of cycling, lifting weights, etc.).

DIAGNOSING PROSTATITIS

Diagnosis is usually made during a DRE (digital rectal exam), where the physician inserts a lubricated, gloved finger into the rectum to feel the prostate, or by examining fluid from the prostate under a microscope. Some doctors use a symptom index questionnaire developed by the National Institutes of Health. Still, diagnosing prostatitis isn't easy, so the most important diagnostic tool your doctor has is you and your detailed descriptions of your symptoms.

Prostatitis is not considered a serious disease, and it doesn't lead to cancer. But it's painful, extremely inconvenient, and sometimes difficult to cure. There are a number of treatment options that usually provide relief. These include antibiotics, anti-inflammatories, and surgery.

BPH (BENIGN PROSTATIC HYPERPLASIA)
BPH, sometimes called "prostate enlargement," is one of the most common conditions among aging men. BPH is caused when an age-related gradual enlargement of the prostate gland squeezes the urethra. Half of men between the ages of 50 and 60 will develop it, and by the age of 70 or 80, about 90 percent will have experienced BPH symptoms, which may include:

- Frequent, often-urgent need to urinate, especially at night
- Need to strain or push to get the urine flowing
- Inability to completely empty the bladder
- Dribbling or leaking after urination
- Weak urine stream

Because male urinary symptoms can also be caused by more serious conditions, such as prostate cancer, it's important to see your doctor to determine the cause of your symptoms.

BPH symptoms vary with the individual. Since the prostate gland continues to grow in most older men, their symptoms may get worse with time. BPH doesn't usually interfere with sexual function, although it can. There is no connection between BPH and cancer. However, if left untreated, the condition can cause bladder infections and kidney stones, and in some cases, permanent bladder and/or kidney damage.

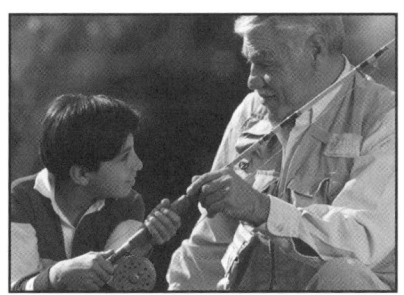

There are three factors that increase your risk of developing BPH:

- Age: Starting at age 45, the risk of developing BPH increases.
- Family history: If any immediate blood relative had BPH, you are more likely to develop the condition.
- Some research indicates that medical conditions such as obesity may contribute to the development of BPH.

Fortunately, the risk of developing uncomfortable BPH symptoms can almost be completely eliminated by diagnosing the condition early. To do that, your doctor may order tests to measure how quickly urine flows from the bladder, and he may do ultrasound or x-ray examinations of the bladder, kidneys, urethra and prostate. He will probably also order a PSA (prostate specific antigen) test. This blood test is often used to diagnose and monitor BPH and to help rule out prostate cancer. (For more information on the PSA test, see the prostate cancer section.)

TREATING BPH
If you are diagnosed with BPH, your doctor has a number of options to choose from.

Watchful Waiting
Watchful waiting means keeping an eye on the BPH symptoms without receiving any form of treatment. For men with minimal to mild BPH symptoms that do not interfere with daily routines, this may be a preferred choice. As part of watchful waiting, men continue to have annual examinations to determine whether their symptoms change over time.

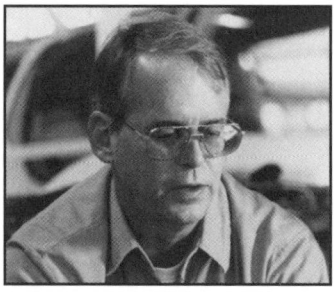

Medications
Drugs called alpha-blockers are the most common treatment prescribed to manage BPH symptoms. By relaxing the muscles around the prostate so that there is less pressure on the urethra, alpha-blockers usually work quickly to improve urinary flow. Common side effects can include stomach or intestinal problems, a stuffy nose, headache, dizziness, tiredness, a drop in blood pressure and ejaculatory problems. Alpha-blockers include Cardura® (doxazosin mesylate), Flomax® (tamsulosin hydrochloride), Hytrin® (terazosin hydrochloride) and Uroxatral® (alfuzosin hydrochloride). *

Another type of drug, known as a 5-alpha-reductase inhibitor, is also sometimes prescribed. Designed to shrink the prostate gland, it may take three to six months to effectively relieve symptoms. Side effects may include an inability to achieve an erection, decreased sexual desire and a reduced amount of semen. Examples of 5-alpha reductase inhibitors are Avodart™ (dutasteride) and Proscar® (finasteride). **

No matter what kind of drug is prescribed, patients and physicians need to be aware of potential drug interactions with treatments used to manage other conditions common among aging men, such as erectile dysfunction and hypertension.

Surgical Treatments
Surgery is typically used only in those patients with major BPH complications such as frequent urinary tract infections or bladder stones. There are several non-surgical approaches that use heat therapy to reduce the size of the prostate, thereby widening the urethra through which urine flows. These heat treatments include microwave therapy, radiofrequency therapy, electrovaporization and laser therapy. In the most extreme cases, open surgery may be required.

Surgery treats BPH symptoms by reducing the size of the prostate, but it does not prevent the cause of the disorder; surgery might need to be repeated within a few years. Side effects of surgery may include urgency and frequency of urination for some period after surgery, difficulty in achieving an erection, blood in your urine, inability to hold your urine (incontinence) or a narrowing of the urethra (scarring).

Cardura is a registered trademark of Pfizer Inc.
Flomax is a registered trademark of Astellas Pharma
Hytrin is a registered trademark of Abbott Laboratories
Uroxatral is a registered trademark of Sanofi Synthelabo, Inc.
***Avodart is a trademark of GlaxoSmithKline*
Proscar is a registered trademark of Merck and Co., Inc.

PROSTATE CANCER
Prostate cancer is the most common cancer in men and the second leading killer of men behind lung cancer. Prostate cancer generally grows slowly and most men die with prostate cancer rather than from it (meaning that they die of some other cause). Still, prostate cancer kills approximately 30,000 men each year. But detected early, it can be cured.

Prostate and skin cancer continue to be the most common cancers in American men.

In its early stages, prostate cancer has no apparent symptoms. However, as the disease progresses, the patient may develop symptoms that are the same as for prostatitis and/or BPH (see above). Additional symptoms include:

- Chronic pain in the hips, thighs, or lower back.
- Blood in the urine or semen.

The lack of early symptoms and the overlap of symptoms with non-cancerous conditions make prostate cancer difficult to diagnose. That's why it's essential that you get screened regularly. (See Appendix B for an age-adjusted schedule.)

RISK FACTORS
There are a handful of factors that could put you at risk of developing prostate cancer:

- **Age:** The risk increases for men age 40 or over with a family history of prostate cancer and African-American men. It increases for men over age 50 otherwise. Prostate cancer is most often diagnosed in men over the age of 65, but it is becoming more common in men between the ages of 55 and 65.
- **Family history:** Your risk of developing prostate cancer is doubled if your father, brother or close male blood relative has had the disease.
- **Race:** African-Americans have the highest rate of prostate cancer in the world, at least twice as high as white men.
- **Diet:** Eating a diet low in fiber and high in fat and red meat, has been shown to increase prostate cancer risk.

If you don't have any symptoms, prostate cancer is often discovered during a regularly scheduled checkup with a DRE and a blood test for PSA (prostate specific antigen), which is often an indicator of prostate-related problems. An abnormal test may mean that you need more testing. These include:

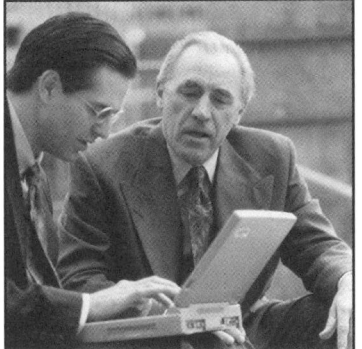

- **Urinalysis:** Often used to rule out BPH or prostatitis.
- **Imaging:** Ultrasound uses sound waves to produce an image of the prostate. MRI and CT scans use computers to produce images. Also, bone scanning can look for prostate cancer that might have spread to the skeletal system.
- **Biopsy:** Taking a number of small pieces of prostate tissue following local anesthesia and examining them under a microscope. This is performed using trans-rectal ultrasound.
- **Lymph node biopsy:** Examination of small samples from the lymph nodes can determine whether the prostate cancer has spread to other parts of the body.

TREATING PROSTATE CANCER
There are a number of options in treating early-stage prostate cancer:

- **Complete surgical removal of the prostate.** Side effects include urinary incontinence (bladder control problems) that can last for weeks, and erectile dysfunction. Options include:
    - Nerve-sparing retropubic radical prostatectomy (NS-RRP).
    - Radical perineal prostatectomy (RPP).
    - Robotic and/or laparoscopic prostatectomy.
    - Nonnerve sparing wide excision radical prostatectomy (RP).
- **Radiation therapy.** There are two options:
    - **High-powered x-rays** are used to kill the cancer cells. Side effects include reduced sexual function, urinary troubles, intestinal difficulty, loss of appetite and hair.
    - **Radioactive seeds.** Your doctor will use a special needle to implant 80 to 120 pellets the size of a grain of rice directly into the prostate. There are fewer sexual side effects but more urinary ones, and there can be damage to the rectum and lower intestines.
- **Hormone therapy.** Because the male sex hormone, testosterone, stimulates cancer cells to grow, you can take drugs to block testosterone production. Hormone therapy is usually not a cure, it's just a way of stopping the tumor from growing. Side effects include breast enlargement, reduced sex drive, weight gain and reduction in muscle mass. One side effect of hormone therapy may be a reduction in testosterone (hypogonadism) which may lead to osteoporosis, which reduces bone mass and may lead to increased risk of bone fractures.
- **Cryosurgery (also called cryotherapy).** This treatment involves freezing the prostate gland in order to destroy the cancer within it. Cryosurgery is an FDA-approved treatment for localized and locally recurrent prostate cancer. It may cause more sexual side effects than other local therapies, but if you're interested, ask your doctor for more information.
- **Observation.** This can be a good option if your doctor believes your cancer is growing very slowly and won't spread to other parts of the body. The advantages are that you avoid all the risks associated with the various treatment options above. Disadvantages are that you'll need regular monitoring in case something changes for the worse. This is also called "watchful waiting" or "active surveillance."

"Prostate cancer can be devastating to an individual, but does not affect men in isolation. It also has, often overlooked, effects on wives, partners, and entire families. We promote regular screenings and early detection of the disease in order to help ensure the best chance of recovery and highest quality of life."

Theresa Morrow, Women Against Prostate Cancer

PREVENTION

- Get your prostate checked yearly after age 40.
- Eat right. Studies show that people who eat a high fat diet have a greater risk of developing prostate cancer. On the other hand, fiber, soy protein, fruits, and cooked tomatoes have all been shown to reduce risk.
- Watch your weight. Obesity may be a contributing factor to a number of cancers, including prostate.
- Exercise regularly.
- Don't smoke.
- Limit alcohol and avoid caffeine.
- Drink a lot of water. This can help flush out your bladder. Urine should be almost clear.
- Have regular sex.
- Consult your doctor about other prevention tips.

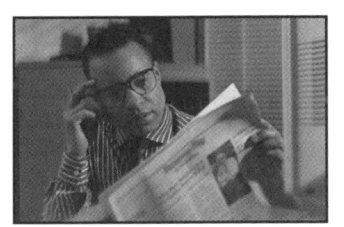

CARDIOVASCULAR SYSTEM

Approximately 450,000 men die of cardiovascular disease each year.

Cardiovascular disease is a blanket term that includes three major types of diseases of the heart and blood vessels: hypertension (high blood pressure), coronary heart disease, and stroke. Over 32 million American men suffer from one or more of these conditions, and every year just under half a million of them die of cardiovascular disease—more than cancer, lung disease, accidents and diabetes combined. Compared to white men, African-American men are more likely to die of cardiovascular disease and Latino men are less likely.

> "The genders are taught to deal with fear and pain differently. When a boy is eight years old and he skins his knee, he is told brave boys don't cry. When he is a teenager playing high school football and gets hurt, they tell him to take it for the team. So when he is 50 years old and having chest pain, he'll say it's just indigestion."
> *Jean Bonhomme, MD, MPH, Men's Health Network*

There are a number of factors that contribute to your likelihood of developing some kind of cardiovascular disease. If any of the following are true about you, make an appointment to see your doctor today:

- An immediate family member was diagnosed with hypertension or some other kind of heart condition before age 55.
- You are African-American.
- You get little or no exercise.
- You are obese.
- You eat a diet high in salt.
- You have high cholesterol (see page 34).
- You smoke. If you do, you are 2-4 times more likely to develop heart disease than a nonsmoker.
- You have high blood pressure.
- You're under a lot of stress.
- You have more than two alcoholic drinks every day.
- You drink a lot of coffee (not decaf).
- You have diabetes (see page 39). More than 80 percent of people with diabetes die of some kind of cardiovascular disease.
- You're taking medication that affects blood pressure. These include Ritalin (for ADD), steroids, migraine medications, any over-the-counter drugs that contain pseudoephedrine, and any medication that contains stimulants such as caffeine.
- You're 45 or older.

CARDIOVASCULAR SYSTEM

Naturally, there's nothing you can do about your age, family history or ethnic background. But there's plenty you can do about all the other risk factors. Let's take a look at each type of cardiovascular disease in detail.

HYPERTENSION/HIGH BLOOD PRESSURE

Blood pressure is a measurement of how hard your blood pushes against the walls of your blood vessels as it flows through your body. The higher the pressure, the harder your heart has to work to do its job. Your blood pressure rises and falls throughout the day, and that's perfectly normal. If you exercise, for example, or win the lottery, or nearly get run over by a car, your blood pressure will go up. But after you've had a chance to catch your breath, it returns to normal.

However, at least a quarter of American men have consistently high blood pressure, which puts a continual strain on the heart and blood vessels and increases the risk of damage to the heart, eyes, kidneys and other organs, and increases the risk of having a heart attack or a stroke.

The good news is that high blood pressure can be treated easily and safely. The bad news is that high blood pressure causes no obvious symptoms; millions of people don't even know they have it.

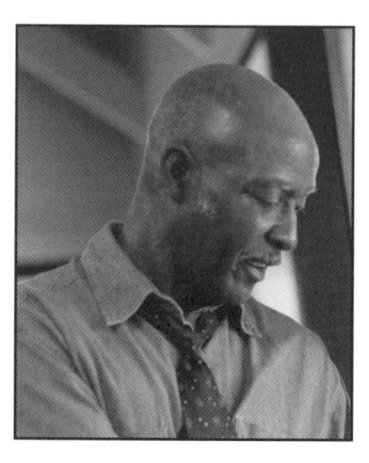

DIAGNOSING AND TREATING HIGH BLOOD PRESSURE

Diagnosing high blood pressure is easy—all you have to do is have your blood pressure checked regularly. However, because men are less likely than women to visit their doctors, they're also less likely to be aware of their blood pressure levels.

In the majority of cases, the causes of high blood pressure are unknown. You can have high blood pressure for years and not know it. It is called the "silent killer." In a percentage of cases, it's caused by taking medication that affects blood pressure or by a chronic medical condition.

CHOLESTEROL

Despite all the negative things people say about cholesterol, the fact is that you couldn't live without it. Cholesterol helps build the walls of every cell in your body; it's involved in making hormones, which send messages throughout your body; and it helps you digest your food.

It's possible, however, to get too much of a good thing. When your body produces more cholesterol than you need, the excess gets into your bloodstream, where it begins to clog your blood vessels. That, in turn, increases your risk of heart disease and stroke.

Besides making your own cholesterol, you get more from the foods you eat. It's found only in animal-based products such as meat, chicken, fish, eggs, milk, and cheese. And while non-animal plant foods don't contain cholesterol, some, such as nuts, oils, and avocados, contain saturated fats, which your body converts into cholesterol during digestion.

What's your cholesterol level?
To measure your cholesterol level, you'll need a blood test. When you look at the results, you'll see that there are actually two different kinds of cholesterol:

- **LDL (low-density lipoprotein)**, often called the "bad" cholesterol, this is the stuff that clogs the blood vessels. An LDL score of 100 or less is considered optimal while a score of 130 or more means you're at risk of developing heart disease.
- **HDL (high-density lipoprotein)**, the "good" cholesterol because it actually removes the LDL. A score of 40 or less may increase the risk of heart disease while a score of 60 or more is good and indicates a lowered risk of heart disease.

Ideally, you want your total cholesterol—the LDL number plus the HDL number—below 200. 200 to 239 is considered moderately high; 240 and above is high.

If your doctor says your cholesterol is too high, you have several options:

- **Make lifestyle changes.** This means eating less saturated fat and high-cholesterol foods like meat, eggs, and dairy products. It also means getting more exercise.
- **Take medication.** Your doctor can prescribe one of several drugs that have been proven to lower cholesterol.

CORONARY HEART DISEASE
Heart disease is the leading killer of men in the United States, causing almost half a million deaths each year. There are two main types of heart disease:

- **Heart attack.** The arteries that supply blood to the heart get blocked, cutting off its oxygen supply. Without oxygen, parts of the heart die and it malfunctions.
- **Angina.** Chest pain caused by a reduced blood supply to the heart.
- **Congestive heart failure.** The heart can't pump enough blood.

The main culprit behind these conditions is atherosclerosis, which is the gradual buildup of plaque on the inside of the arteries. This plaque is made up of cholesterol, calcium, and normal cellular waste products. The more plaque, the less blood can flow to the heart and other organs.

But the real danger occurs when the plaque ruptures, causing blood clots. If a blood clot blocks an artery, no blood can get through. If this happens near the heart, a heart attack occurs. If it happens near the brain, a stroke occurs (see page 36).

HEART ATTACK

Most heart attacks are caused by a blood clot resulting from ruptured plaque. Men suffer heart attacks an average of 10 years younger than women do, and they're more likely to die of heart disease than women of the same age. The death rate for African-American men is even higher than it is for whites. Sadly, half of the men who die of heart disease weren't even aware that they had a problem.

If you experience any of the following, contact your doctor immediately:

- Pressure or squeezing in the center of the chest
- Pain that spreads over the shoulders, neck, and arms
- Increased heartbeat
- Sweating
- Nausea
- Shortness of breath
- Irregular heart beat

ANGINA

About 7 million men have this condition. Symptoms (pressure in the chest or down the left arm) are temporary—lasting 15 minutes or less. Most people who have angina describe their symptoms as "uncomfortable," as opposed to "painful."

If you have any symptoms of angina, consider yourself lucky (better to have a little pain and get treatment, than no symptoms and a sudden heart attack), and make an appointment to see your doctor immediately.

CONGESTIVE HEART FAILURE

Congestive heart failure—a reduction in the heart's pumping capacity—is usually a condition that starts many years before it's ever noticed and gradually worsens over time. The heart tries to compensate for lost capacity by getting bigger and by pumping faster. In order to make sure that the most important organs—the heart and the brain—have adequate blood supply, the body diverts blood away from other less-important organs. At the same time, the body starts retaining fluids, which back up into the lungs and other parts of the body.

Over 2 million men currently suffer from heart failure and about 300,000 more are diagnosed each year. It is the leading cause of hospitalization in people 65 and older. Symptoms include shortness of breath, fatigue, dizziness, low blood pressure, sudden large weight gain, frequent nighttime urination, and swelling of the lower legs and ankles.

There is no cure for heart failure. However, if you manage it correctly, you can live a long, healthy, productive life.

STROKE

When one of the blood vessels that keep the brain supplied with oxygen gets blocked or bursts, the brain doesn't get the oxygen it needs to function. Nerve cells start dying within a minute, and as they die, the functions they controlled stop working. Although your body replaces dead cells everywhere else in your body, brain cells aren't replaced, which means that any damage done by a stroke is permanent.

The most common side effects of a stroke are numbness or inability to move the arm or leg or facial muscles on one side of the body, depression, visual problems, and difficulty speaking or understanding speech.

Warning signs of a stroke come on suddenly and unexpectedly and include:

- Confusion, or difficulty speaking or understanding (speech).
- Numbness or difficulty controlling one side of the face or one side of the body.
- Vision problems.
- Difficulty walking or loss of balance, or trouble holding onto things.
- Severe unexplained headache.

If you notice any of these symptoms in yourself or anyone around you, call 911 or your local emergency number immediately. Again, the damage caused by a stroke is permanent and gets worse with each second.

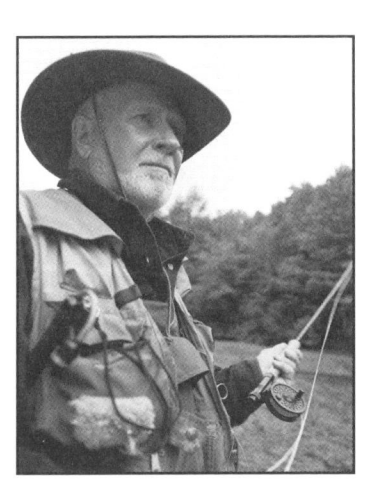

TREATING AND PREVENTING CARDIOVASCULAR DISEASE

If your doctor believes that you have any type of cardiovascular disease or are at risk of developing one or more, he'll probably tell you to do one or more of the following:

- Take aspirin every day. Talk to your doctor first, though, and don't exceed the dose he suggests. Aspirin prevents blood clots which can trigger heart attacks.
- Have regular physicals (see Appendix B for a complete schedule) and make sure to tell your doctors about any uncomfortable symptoms especially chest pain and shortness of breath while resting.
- Lose weight. As your weight increases, so does your blood pressure. As important as your weight is where you store the fat. If you carry your weight around your middle, you have a higher risk than if you carry it around the hips and thighs. Losing weight will have an immediate effect on your blood pressure.
- Get into a regular exercise routine. Being active cuts your risk of developing high blood pressure by 25 to 50 percent.
- Limit your alcohol intake to two drinks a day or less.
- Limit your non-decaf coffee consumption to two cups a day.
- Reduce stress.
- Quit smoking. There is no safe level of smoking. Every cigarette does damage.
- Change your diet (see page 9). Look for "very low sodium" or "sodium free" on labels, avoid saturated fats and hydrogenated oils, eat more whole

grains, eat fish twice a week or take an Omega-3 supplement, limit red meat and eggs, and eat more garlic and onions, which have been shown to reduce blood pressure.
- Get a pet. Research has shown that petting animals, and even looking at fish in an aquarium lowers blood pressure.
- Brush your teeth. Some interesting recent research suggests that there may be a connection between gum disease and an increased risk for heart disease and stroke.

In addition, your doctor might also prescribe some drugs to lower your blood pressure or cholesterol. If he does, be sure to tell him about all other medications or over-the-counter drugs you take, since some combinations of drugs can cause trouble. And don't stop taking the medication—even if you're feeling great—unless your doctor advises you to.

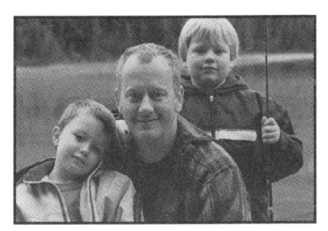

DIABETES

Diabetes is a very serious condition that affects your body's ability to turn what you eat into the energy your body needs to function. Diabetes contributes to the deaths of over 200,000 Americans every year. Also, it is a leading cause of heart disease, strokes, kidney failure, blindness and amputations. People with diabetes are more than twice as likely to develop heart disease or die from a heart attack than people without diabetes.

> **Diabetes is a leading cause of heart disease, strokes, kidney failure, blindness and amputations.**

Everything you eat and drink is digested in your stomach and most of it broken down into sugar molecules called glucose. Glucose gets absorbed into your bloodstream and is transported to cells in every part of your body. A hormone called insulin unlocks the cells and allows the glucose to enter, where it provides the fuel that keeps the cells alive and working.

Diabetes is what happens if your body doesn't produce enough insulin to take glucose out of your bloodstream, or if your cells don't respond to insulin's attempts to unlock them. The result is an excess of sugar in the bloodstream, which can cause damage to every major system in your body.

Over 18 million Americans have diabetes. Latinos are much more likely to develop diabetes than whites, and African-Americans are about 60 percent more likely. In addition, over 40 million Americans have what's called pre-diabetes, which means they have blood glucose levels that are higher than normal, but not quite high enough to be diagnosed as diabetic. A large percentage of people with pre-diabetes eventually develop diabetes.

There are two major types of diabetes:

- **Type 1**, where the body produces little or no insulin. Type 1 accounts for only 5 to 10 percent of cases and is most common among children. It requires daily injections of insulin.
- **Type 2**, where the body produces at least some insulin, but cells don't respond to it. Type 2 accounts for 90 to 95 percent of cases. Type 2 diabetes is most common among people over 40 who are overweight. But as Americans get fatter and get less exercise, Type 2 diabetes is becoming more common among children as well. Unfortunately, over 5 million people have this type of diabetes and don't know it.

DIAGNOSING DIABETES

Type 1 diabetes develops very quickly—usually over a few days or weeks—and the symptoms are often severe. These include:

- Frequent urination and larger-than-normal amounts of urine, especially at night.
- Dry mouth and excessive thirst.
- Sudden feeling of fatigue.
- Unexplained weight loss.
- Blurry vision.

Type 2 diabetes develops much more slowly and the symptoms are much less noticeable. In fact, by the time people are diagnosed with Type 2 diabetes, they've had the disease for an average of over five years without knowing it. Many of the early symptoms of Type 2 diabetes are the same as for Type 1, but the difference is that they develop so slowly that they often go unnoticed. Other symptoms include:

- Tingling or numbness of the hands and feet.
- Cuts and scrapes that take a long time to heal.
- Urinary tract infections.
- Impotence or erectile dysfunction (see page 21 for more).

Because the symptoms of Type 2 diabetes are so hard to recognize, the diagnosis is often only made during a routine medical checkup. Pre-diabetes, which has no visible symptoms at all, is even harder to diagnose. So if you are experiencing any of the symptoms above or any of the risk factors listed below, schedule an exam right now. If your doctor suspects that you may have diabetes or pre-diabetes, he'll order several blood tests to measure the glucose levels in your blood and your body's ability to process it.

Risk factors for diabetes and pre-diabetes include:

- Being 45 or older.
- Being overweight, especially if you carry your weight around the middle as opposed to around your hips.
- Having a parent, brother or sister with Type 2 diabetes.
- Belonging to a high-risk ethnic group (African-American, Latino, Asian-American, Pacific Islander, American Indian).
- Exercising fewer than two times per week.
- Having high blood pressure and/or high cholesterol.

LIVING WITH AND PREVENTING DIABETES

There is no cure for diabetes, however, it can be managed and treated. And about 90 percent of the time, diabetes can be prevented before it starts. The keys to prevention and treatment are basic:

- Lose weight.
- Control your blood pressure.
- Get more exercise.
- Eat a healthy, balanced diet.

If you're being treated for diabetes, you'll see your doctor every few months. He may prescribe some medication, but there are limits to what he can do. Ultimately, it's up to you: you'll need to monitor your glucose levels at home, take your medication exactly the way you're supposed to, keep all of your medical appointments, and make the necessary lifestyle changes.

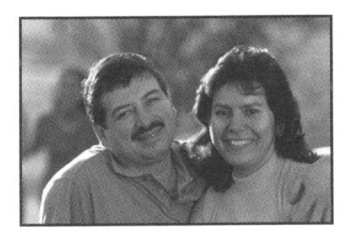

CANCER

Over 700,000 men are diagnosed with cancer each year and nearly 300,000 die of it. Over the course of a lifetime, half of all men will get cancer at least once. Cancer can strike anyone, at any age, but the majority of cases happen to people 55 and over.

Approximately 700,000 men are diagnosed with cancer each year and nearly 300,000 die of it.

The saddest part about all of this is that most of these cancers and deaths are preventable. At least one-third of cancer deaths are caused by smoking, and another one-third may be caused by poor diet and/or lack of exercise.

The two keys to beating cancer are early detection and reducing risk.

RISK FACTORS
If any of the following are true, you are at risk of developing cancer. It doesn't mean you will, just that you should be in close contact with your doctor.

- You smoke (cigarettes, pipes, or cigars) or chew tobacco.
- You drink more than two alcoholic drinks per day.
- You have a family history of cancer.
- You have had cancer in the past.
- You are 55 or older.
- You get little or no exercise.
- You eat a high-fat, low-fiber diet.
- You are African-American.

EARLY DETECTION
You can't detect cancers if you don't know what to look for. Below are a number of symptoms that could be indicators. Many of them could be caused by other conditions, but you should notify your doctor if you notice anything unusual or abnormal.

- Lumps that you can feel through the skin.
- Sores that don't heal.
- Changes in the size, color, or texture of a wart or mole.
- Blood in the urine, stool, or saliva.
- A cough, sore throat, hoarseness, or trouble swallowing that won't go away.
- Persistent back ache.
- Unexpected weight loss.
- Unexplained pain.
- Pressure or tenderness in the chest.
- Unusual bleeding.
- Chronic nausea or gas.
- Fever that lasts more than a few days.

PREVENTING CANCER

Even with early detection and knowledge of the risk factors, there's no way to guarantee that you'll never get cancer. But there are a number of steps you can take that will go a long way toward minimizing your chances.

According to the American Cancer Society, the approximate lifetime risk of developing cancer is 1-in-2 for men and 1-in-3 for women.

- Don't smoke. Smoking causes 90 percent of lung cancers and greatly increases the risk of cancers of the mouth, kidney, bladder, pancreas and esophagus.
- Limit alcohol to two drinks a day maximum.
- Limit your exposure to sunlight. A little bit of exposure will stimulate your body to produce vitamin D, which researchers think may reduce the risk of a number of cancers. But too much can cause skin cancer. Between 10 am and 3 pm—the hottest part of the day—try to stay indoors as much as possible. When you do go out, always wear sunscreen with SPF (sunscreen protection factor) 25 or greater. If you don't have sunscreen, wear a hat or stay in the shade as much as possible. Having fair skin or having had severe sunburn in childhood greatly increases the risk of developing skin cancer.
- Eat a low-fat, high fiber diet with lots of fruits, vegetables, and whole grains. High-fat, low-fiber diets are at least partly responsible for most colorectal cancers. They also increase the risk of pancreatic and bladder cancers.
- Limit foods that are smoked, salted, pickled, or high in nitrates (such as hot dogs and luncheon meats). These foods are associated with increased risk of stomach cancer.
- Limit your exposure to PVCs (poly vinyl chloride), tar and creosote (a dark brown or black flammable tar deposited from wood smoke on chimney walls). These are linked with a number of cancers, including cancer of the liver and skin.
- Spend some time getting to know yourself and your body. See your physician if you notice any significant changes.
- Get screened as recommended in Appendix B. These tests are designed to detect certain types of cancer (such as colon, bladder, kidney, testicles, prostate) in their earliest stages. Caught early, these cancers can be treated successfully.
- Take aspirin. Some recent research indicates that people who took aspirin 16 times a month or more were 40 percent less likely to get cancer of the esophagus, stomach, rectum, or colon than those who didn't take aspirin at all.

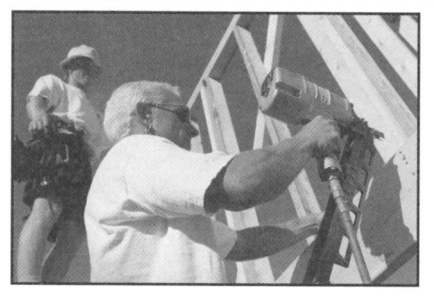

See page 29 for information on prostate cancer
See page 45 for information on testicular cancer

Can Men Get Breast Cancer? Absolutely.

Although breast cancer is usually thought of as a women's disease, about 1 percent of breast cancers occur in men. No less a man than Richard Roundtree, who played Shaft in the 1970s movie has been diagnosed with breast cancer. The most common early symptom is a lump in the breast, usually right underneath the nipple. More advanced symptoms include a bloody discharge from the nipple or a retraction of the nipple. A lot of men who notice symptoms like these put off going to the doctor because they believe that a "real man" wouldn't get breast cancer. That kind of attitude could kill you. So if you notice either of these symptoms, or you just have a feeling that something isn't right, schedule a medical appointment right away.

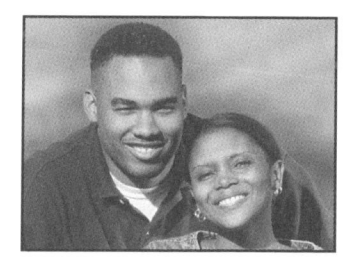

TESTICULAR CANCER

Testicular cancer is the most common type of cancer in young men ages 15 to 35. Early detection is critical because testicular cancer typically grows quickly and begins to spread to other parts of the body just a few months after the first symptoms appear. But treated early, it is almost 100 percent curable.

Testicular cancer, caught and treated early, is almost 100 percent curable.

RISK FACTORS
There are several factors that increase men's risk of developing testicular cancer:

- **Age.** Most common in men 15 to 35, but can strike any man at any age.
- **Undescended testicle(s)**, even if they were brought to normal position as a child.
- **Family history** of testicular cancer.
- **Being Caucasian.** White men are slightly more likely to develop testicular cancer than Hispanics, twice as likely as Asian-Americans, and five to ten times more likely than African-Americans.
- **Diet.** Several recent studies have found that eating a lot of cheese and other dairy products increases the risk of developing testicular cancer. Luncheon meats and a high-red-meat/low-fruit diet also increases the risk.

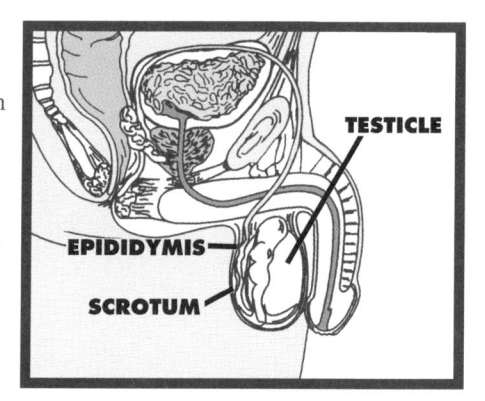

EARLY DETECTION
The best way to identify symptoms is to do a simple, three-minute self-exam once a month beginning on your 15th birthday. Here's how to do the exam:

- Get into the shower or a warm bath. Heat causes the scrotum skin to relax, making the exam easier.
- Soap up. Fingers glide over soapy skin, making it easier to concentrate on the texture underneath.
- Using both hands, slowly roll each testicle between the thumb and fingers, applying slight pressure. It's completely normal to find that one testicle may be slightly larger.
- Try to find hard, pea-sized, painless bumps in the testicles ("balls") themselves.

TESTICULAR CANCER

- Ignore the epididymis. The epididymis is a cord-like structure on the top and back of the testicle that stores and transports the sperm.
- See your doctor promptly if you feel or see anything suspicious. Also tell your doctor if you experience any pain or a heavy feeling in either testicle.

By doing these exams regularly, you'll learn what a normal testicle feels like. And that will make it much easier to know if something changes.

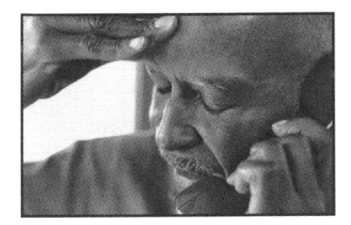

EMOTIONAL HEALTH AND WELL-BEING

> Depression is under-diagnosed in men. Men are over four times more likely than women to commit suicide.

Your emotional and mental heath have an effect on everything in your life, from your relationships with others and your career successes to how long you live. In this chapter, we'll talk about some of the ways your emotions affect your physical health.

STRESS

Stress is an unavoidable fact of life, and all of us suffer from it once in a while. There are literally thousands of events or situations (both positive and negative) that can create stress, including:

- **Family:** Birth of a child, death of a relative, marriage, arguments, divorce, moving to a new house, starting a new school.
- **Money:** Going into debt, watching the stock market plummet, private school tuition.
- **Workplace:** Getting a new promotion, not getting a promotion, not feeling appreciated, arguing with your boss or a coworker, pushing yourself too hard.
- **Your body:** Injury, chronic illness, chronic pain, sexual problems, not getting enough sleep, substance abuse, smoking, poor nutrition.
- **Other:** Being stuck in traffic when you're already late, having to make a speech in public.

When you're feeling stressed, your heart beats faster, your blood pressure rises, and your muscles tense. A little bit of stress is actually good for you. It can focus your attention, give you a sudden burst of strength to get out of a dangerous situation, motivate you to succeed, and even stimulate your creativity. After whatever caused the stress has passed, your heart rate returns to normal and you get on with your life.

But when the cause of your stress doesn't go away, it starts eating away at your immune system and increases your risk of developing a number of physical and mental conditions, including:

- Constant fatigue
- Trouble falling or staying asleep
- Headaches and backaches
- Short-term memory loss
- Inability to concentrate
- Feeling out of control
- Eating, drinking, or smoking when nervous
- Anger and irritability
- Irritable bowels
- Back and neck pain
- Sexual problems
- Loss of appetite
- Asthma
- Heart disease
- Diabetes
- Stroke

EMOTIONAL HEALTH AND WELL-BEING

- Paying less attention to your appearance
- Paying less attention to your family
- Stomach ache and indigestion
- Cancer
- Depression

We all have our individual ways of dealing with stress. You might bite your nails or sit staring at your computer for hours. Or you might do something more self-destructive, like smoke, get drunk, drive too fast, or get into fights. Finding effective ways to cope with your stress is vital to your physical and mental health. And the best coping strategies involve making lifestyle changes. Here are a few suggestions:

- **Take care of yourself.** Exercise, eat well, and get plenty of sleep. If you are so stressed out that you can't take care of yourself, you won't be able to take care of the people in your life who are depending on you.
- **Meditate.** Meditation has been shown to lower blood pressure and relieve tension. This can be as simple as setting aside 10 minutes a day to close your eyes, clear your mind, and focus on your breathing.
- **Talk to someone else.** Having a support network of friends or family who can help you makes a huge difference in your ability to cope.
- **Prioritize.** Do the most important things first, save the least important ones for later.
- **Know your limits.** Ask yourself, "What's the worst thing that could happen if I just stopped what I'm doing and walked away?" Your answer might surprise you.
- **Don't self-medicate:** no alcohol, tobacco, or drugs.

DEPRESSION

Depression is one of the most common diseases, affecting over 6 million men in this country. But as common as depression is, it's also one of the most misunderstood diseases. Many people believe, for example, that depression is a normal part of life, something you should just smile and snap out of. It's not nearly that simple.

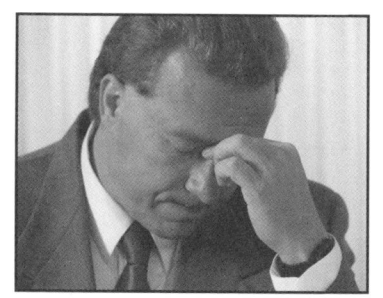

Yes, everyone feels a little down-in-the-dumps once in a while. Maybe you broke up with a girlfriend, or your new car was stolen, or you got passed over for that promotion you'd been counting on. For most people, these feelings pass after a few days.

But if you're depressed, those feelings of sadness or hopelessness or disappointment don't pass. You may become obsessed with negative thoughts and not be able to stop yourself from focusing on things that have gone wrong, feel that you're a burden to others, or that you're a failure.

Depression has a negative impact on the lives of the people who suffer from it and those who love them. It can break up marriages, end friendships, harm parent-child relationships and destroy the depressed person's health. Depression is the leading cause of disability in the U.S., sidelining more people than back problems, heart disease, or injuries.

Although depression is generally considered a mental illness, most depressed men will have both physical and psychological symptoms, including:

- General aches and pains, such as headache, backache, blurred vision, indigestion.
- Constant feelings of sadness or frequent crying.
- A drop in performance on the job or in school.
- Regularly feeling angry, irritable, tense or on edge.
- Withdrawing from people.
- Loss of interest or enjoyment in activities and things you used to like.
- Feelings of guilt for no apparent reason.
- Generalizing problems, meaning that having a problem in one area makes you feel like your whole life is coming apart.
- Change in sleeping patterns—either sleeping more than usual or less.
- Significant weight loss or gain for no particular reason.
- Loss of self-confidence.
- Decreased ability to make decisions or concentrate.
- Difficulty completing daily tasks (such as returning phone calls, paying bills, picking up the kids from school or making dinner).
- Trouble finishing projects or delivering on promises.
- Trouble motivating yourself to do anything.
- Feelings of worthlessness, hopelessness, loneliness, or helplessness.
- Feeling tired and worn down.
- Thoughts of death or suicide.

As devastating as depression can be, the good news is that in most cases it's treatable. Unfortunately most men who have depression don't seek treatment. Some men don't know (or don't want to know) that they have the disease. Other men are afraid of seeming weak or defective if they admit they suffer from depression. And in too many cases, men try to solve their problems by self-medicating with alcohol or drugs.

If you experience any of the above symptoms for more than two weeks, or if you feel that any of these symptoms are interfering with your life, see a doctor right away. Not getting the help you need will only make the problem worse for you and those around you.

CAUSES OF DEPRESSION
In some cases, depression can be caused by an imbalance of chemicals in the brain—specifically a deficit of the chemicals that are responsible for maintaining energy and boosting mood. Having a family member with depression increases your risk, and major life events (such as a divorce, physical disability, bankruptcy or death) can make depression worse.

TREATING DEPRESSION
The sooner you begin to deal with your depression the better. In many cases, mild depression can be dealt with by making lifestyles changes, such as:

EMOTIONAL HEALTH AND WELL-BEING

- Talking to friends or relatives about what's making you depressed.
- Eliminating drugs or alcohol.
- Setting more realistic goals.
- Making sure you get enough sleep and set aside some time for fun activities.
- Exercising regularly.
- Making an attempt to spend time with people and not isolating yourself.

More severe depression requires medical attention, either by taking medication or going through psychotherapy, or some combination of the two. If your doctor does prescribe medication, there are several important things to remember:

- Be patient. Too many men start taking antidepressants but give up after only a week or so, feeling that they've failed. It usually takes two to four weeks (and sometimes as long as eight weeks) before you'll become aware of a change for the better. And sometimes your doctor will have to experiment with two or three drugs before finding the one that works best for you.
- Take the drugs exactly as your doctor prescribes them, and keep taking them until he says to stop. With some you have to start with a low dose and gradually ramp up.
- Don't stop taking the medication until your doctor says to. It's often tempting to stop taking medication once you begin to feel better. But sometimes stopping abruptly can be dangerous.
- Discuss the side effects and possible interactions with other medications that you're taking.

Don't make the mistake of thinking you can cure your problems by taking some medication. In most cases, medication is far more effective when combined with psychotherapy.

SUICIDE RISK
Failing to treat depression can have many devastating consequences, the most serious of which is suicide. There are a number of factors that increase the risk of attempting or succeeding at suicide.

- Being male. Men are four times more likely than women to kill themselves.
- Being a teenager or senior citizen.
- Getting a divorce, particularly if you have children.
- Drug and/or alcohol use.
- Being isolated. People who live alone or who don't have friends are at a higher risk.

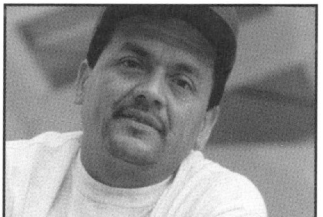

ADDICTION AND SUBSTANCE ABUSE

Cigarette smoke is responsible for over 400,000 deaths every year.

When most people hear the word addict they think of illegal drug use. But there are literally dozens of other kinds of addictions. For example, people can also be addicted to:

- Prescription drugs
- Club drugs
- Alcohol
- Nicotine
- Food
- Sex
- Stealing
- Gambling
- The Internet
- Steroids
- Exercise
- Television
- Work
- Risk-taking
- Sugar

WHAT IS ADDICTION?
It doesn't matter whether the addictive substance or behavior is legal or illegal, all addictions are basically the same: an uncontrollable urge to do something or consume something, regardless of the harm it causes.

When you take drugs or drink alcohol or engage in certain activities, your brain releases chemicals called neurotransmitters that create a wave of positive feelings ranging from pleasure to invincibility. The brain and body enjoy those sensations so much that they "demand" them again, by creating a craving for the same substance or behavior. But this time, it'll take a little bit more to get the same rush.

Over a very short period of time, the neurotransmitters actually make permanent changes to the structure of the brain. Satisfying the cravings becomes more and more important, and not satisfying them causes physical pain. The consequences can be devastating to the addict, his family, his friends and his community. Relationships are destroyed, life savings are spent, people end up in prison, and lives are lost. Men are five times more likely to abuse drugs or alcohol than women.

Of course, not everyone who tries a particular drug or engages in risky behavior becomes an addict. But in many cases even one time use can be harmful or even deadly.

Let's take a look at several of the most common—and most harmful—abused substances. The big three—tobacco, alcohol, and drug abuse—are responsible for one in four deaths in this country.

TOBACCO
Cigarette smoke contains several thousand chemicals, including over 100 that are known poisons, and it's responsible for over 400,000 deaths every year—more than alcohol, cocaine, heroin, AIDS, murder, suicide, and car accidents combined. American Indians smoke cigarettes more than any other racial group.

Even if it doesn't kill you, smoking tobacco decreases your senses of smell and taste, causes a nasty cough, wrinkles your skin, discolors your fingernails, loosens your teeth, makes you depressed, causes erectile dysfunction, weakens your immune system, and exposes everyone around you to the same dangers.

If you thought that smoking a pipe or cigars, or chewing tobacco or snuff is less dangerous, think again. Non-cigarette tobacco use is linked to cancer of the mouth and larynx, as wells as emphysema.

The best way to quit is to join a support group and start using nicotine patches or gum. There are also a number of other options that your doctor may recommend. Stay away from smokers and ask your friends and family to support and encourage you in any way that they can.

Quitting smoking has immediate effects. Less than an hour after your last cigarette, your blood pressure and heart rate begin dropping to normal levels. Within one day, your risk of having a heart attack is already lower. After two days your sense of smell and taste start improving, and after two weeks, your lung function will be much improved—you won't cough as much, you'll be less tired, and less short of breath. Looking down the road, 10 years after you quit, your risk of stroke will be about the same as a non-smoker's, and your risk of developing lung cancer will be half what it was the day you quit.

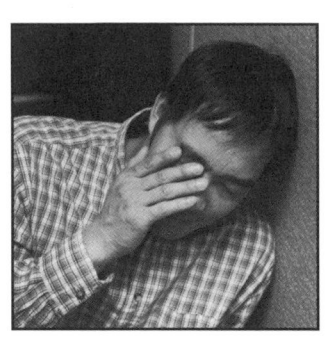

ALCOHOL

In moderate quantities (no more than two drinks per day), alcohol may help reduce the risk of heart disease. Unfortunately, millions of American men (and women) aren't able to keep their alcohol consumption "moderate." The consequences are extremely negative.

Excessive alcohol consumption kills approximately 75,000-85,000 Americans every year, over 70 percent of whom are men. It's also responsible for about one in four hospital stays and is a factor in 60 percent of acts of violence. Alcohol can also cause stomach ulcers and do long-term damage to the liver, brain and heart.

Among ethnic groups, Hispanics are the most likely to be heavy drinkers, followed by whites and African-Americans. African-Americans, however, have the highest death rates of the three groups. African-Americans are also more likely than whites or Hispanics to suffer from alcohol-related liver disease.

What makes alcohol a little different from some of the other addictions is that you don't have to be an alcoholic to have problems with it. Over half of alcohol-related deaths are the result of binge drinking (five or more drinks in one sitting). And while many people have the impression that binging is something only high schoolers and college students do, three-quarters of binge drinking deaths occurred among men over 35.

ADDICTION AND SUBSTANCE ABUSE

DRUG ABUSE
The most commonly used illegal drugs in the US are:

- Marijuana (used by over 14 million people age 12 and over).
- Cocaine, including crack (over 2 million).
- Hallucinogens, such as LSD and mushrooms (1.2 million).
- Club drugs, including ecstasy, GHB, ketamine, and the date rape drug rohypnol (over 5 million).
- Heroin (200,000).

Using any of these drugs, even once, can be risky. At the very least, they slow your reaction time and impair your judgment, which increases the chance that you'll engage in some kind of risky behavior, such as driving while high, having unsafe sex, or consuming even more drugs. Some first-time users may experience vomiting and seizures. At worst, an overdose can result in permanent injury or death.

If you become addicted and use drugs for an extended period, the risks go way up, and include:

- Aggressive, violent or paranoid behavior
- Anxiety
- Depression
- Memory loss
- Lack of interest in the way you look or dress
- Increased risk of getting an STD, including AIDS
- Criminal activity (many addicts steal or rob to get the money to buy their drugs)
- Destroyed family relationships
- Bankruptcy
- Increased heart rate and blood pressure
- Damage to the heart, liver, or kidneys
- Respiratory infection
- Sexual problems
- Stroke
- Coma
- Sudden death

Although most discussions of drug use have focused on the drugs listed above, other drugs and stimulants are commonly abused including prescription drugs (stimulants, sedatives, tranquilizers, and pain killers) and over-the-counter (OTC) items such as cough medicine, glue, paint thinner and nail polish. Over 20 million Americans admit to having used one or more of these legal drugs for non-medical purposes within the past year.

Some people who are addicted to prescription drugs or OTC drugs started taking them for medical purposes on the advice of their health care provider, and became addicted unintentionally. On the other hand, people who abuse glue,

ADDICTION AND SUBSTANCE ABUSE

paint thinner, or cough medicines (which can contain a lot of alcohol), use these products intentionally to get high. Either way, these legal products can be just as addictive as illegal ones, and they can cause just as much short- and long-term damage to the user and his family.

Although drug use is often thought of as a problem of people living in poor, inner-city neighborhoods, drugs affect all parts of our society and have a destructive effect on communities.

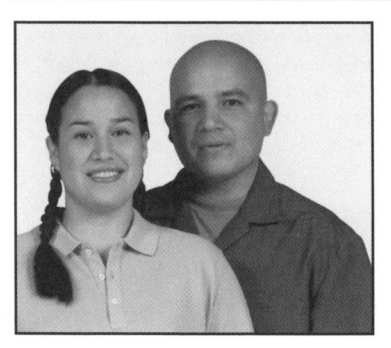

HIDDEN ADDICTIONS
Thirty years ago, almost no one talked about alcoholism. Fifteen years ago, no one talked about cocaine addiction. And until a few years ago, no one had even heard of ecstasy and the other club drugs.

Today everyone knows about the dangers of all these addictions, but there are many others that aren't being talked about. These include compulsive gambling, sex addiction, and Internet addiction.

What separates these addictions from most others is that they involve behavior, not substances. But the effects on the brain are the same and the consequences are often devastating. Let's take a brief look at each one.

Compulsive Gambling
Between five and 15 million Americans from all walks of life are addicted to gambling. Over three-quarters of compulsive gamblers suffer from depression, and they're 20 times more likely than a non-addict to commit suicide. Compulsive gambling is also linked with higher rates of divorce, violence, stealing and child abuse.

Sexual Addiction
Sex addicts compulsively look for and engage in sexual behavior, even when they know it's risky to themselves, their family, or others. Sex addicts can't control their sexual feelings, and they will sacrifice their jobs, their health, and their relationships to satisfy their need for arousal. Sex addicts have higher-than-average rates of broken relationships and divorce, STD, AIDS, financial and legal problems, depression, alcoholism and other substance abuse, and imprisonment.

Internet Addiction
Addicts can get hooked on chat rooms, games, checking email and aimlessly surfing the web, and spend an average of almost 40 hours per week online. Internet addicts may call in sick from work in order to spend more time on the computer. They'll cut back on sleep, eating, homework and spending time with family and children. And like other addicts, they suffer painful withdrawal if they're away from the computer for even a few hours.

ADDICTION AND SUBSTANCE ABUSE

TREATING ADDICTIONS

If you're addicted to any illegal or legal drug and want to get clean, the first thing you need to do is admit that you have a problem. But that's harder than it sounds, since most addicts are in denial or tell themselves that they "can quit anytime."

Once you can be honest with yourself, you need to get help. Breaking an addiction alone is almost impossible. So talk with your doctor about getting into a rehab program. Don't worry that he'll turn you in—he won't.

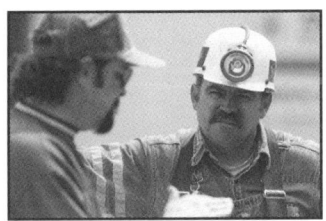

ACCIDENT PREVENTION AND SAFETY

Accidents are the #1 cause of death for men under age 44.

With all the attention paid to cancer, stroke, heart disease, and diabetes, we almost never hear about another men's health crisis: accidents. Accidents are one of the top five killers of men and for those under age 44, they're the number one cause of death. Men are far more likely than women to be injured or killed in an accident, largely because men tend to engage in riskier behavior. And American-Indian men are significantly more likely than other men to die from accidents. Let's talk about the major types of accidents and how to prevent them.

MOTOR VEHICLE CRASHES

Car crashes are the leading cause of accidental death among men. Men are more likely to be involved in a fatal crash than women. While you can't control what other drivers do, there are a number of steps you can take to reduce accidents:

- Always wear your seatbelt, even on short trips.
- Follow posted speed limits.
- Don't drive after drinking or when you're tired.
- Don't drive with someone else who's intoxicated or exhausted.
- Always wear a helmet when riding a motorcycle, bicycle or skateboard.

ACCIDENTAL POISONING

This is the second leading cause of accidental death. Men are more than twice as likely as women to die from poisoning. You should keep the national poison control number **(1-800-222-1222)** posted near your telephone or programmed into your speed dial. Here's what else you can do to reduce your risk:

- Install smoke and carbon monoxide detectors in your home. Replace the batteries twice a year.
- Carefully follow the instructions on household cleaning products. Mixing bleach and ammonia, for example, produces a toxic gas.
- If you're using chemicals, be sure you've got plenty of ventilation.
- Take prescription medication exactly as your doctor prescribes, and follow directions on non-prescription drugs.

FALLS

Accidental falls are the leading cause of injury and injury-related death among those over 65.

- Stay active. Physical activity helps preserve your balance.
- Use appropriate lighting. Not being able to see in the dark can lead to tripping and falls.
- Install railings on stairways and next to bathtubs and showers.
- Put non-skid pads underneath rugs and carpets.

ACCIDENT PREVENTION AND SAFETY

- Use ladders safely.
- Starting at age 60, get screened for osteoporosis. See the screening and checkup guidelines in Appendix B.

WORKPLACE ACCIDENTS

Over 90 percent of people who die on the job are men. That's largely because men are much more likely than women to work in high-risk jobs, such as construction, mining, hazardous materials and roofing.

- Take every safety precaution. That means wearing hard hats, seat belts, safety harnesses, masks, eye protection, and asking for help when you need it.
- Take extra care when handling chemicals. Many are linked with asthma, cancer and infertility.

GUNS

The easiest way to prevent accidental shootings is to not keep firearms in your home. But if you do, be sure to:

- Keep guns unloaded and securely locked.
- Keep ammunition in a separate location.
- Keep guns and ammunition in a gun safe or secure gun locker.
- Be especially careful when cleaning guns—this is when many gun accidents happen.

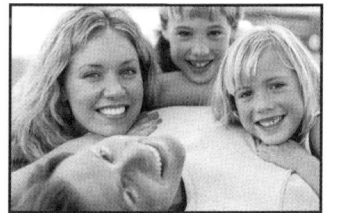

FATHERHOOD

Although one generally doesn't think of being a dad as a health issue, there's no question that it is.

IT'S GOOD FOR YOU

Many men find that becoming a father gives their life new meaning. It also provides a reason to make positive changes in their lives, such as quitting smoking and drinking, driving more carefully, eating better, getting more exercise, and managing stress. Overall, men who are actively involved in their children's lives tend to be healthier, have more fulfilling careers and marriages, and live longer.

Children are more likely to do well academically, to participate in extracurricular activities, and to enjoy school and are less likely to have ever repeated a grade or to have been suspended or expelled if their fathers have high as opposed to low involvement in their schools.
National Center For Education Statistics

IT'S GOOD FOR YOUR CHILDREN

Research shows that children with involved fathers do better in school, are more likely to graduate high school, have more friends, have fewer psychological problems, and are less likely to smoke, abuse drugs or alcohol, engage in risky behavior, start having sex early, or become teen parents.

STAYING INVOLVED AFTER DIVORCE OR SEPARATION

If you're divorced or never married, being an involved dad is critical. You may not be able to see your children as often as you'd like, but that doesn't mean you're not important to them. So never miss a chance to spend time with your child. Being a frequent and regular presence in their lives will give them the same benefits outlined above. And be sure to get involved in your children's school. Children are more likely to get A's in school, to enjoy school, and to participate in extracurricular activities if their nonresident fathers are involved in their schools, according to the U.S. Department of Education.

BEING A GOOD ROLE MODEL

One of the most important ways dads improve their children's physical and psychological health is by setting a good example. Boys learn from their fathers what it means to be a man in our society. With a good role model, they will learn how to treat women properly, and they will learn that you don't have to be a tough guy to be a man.

Don't underestimate your importance as a role model for your daughters. As the first man in her life, you influence her in many ways. How you treat your wife sets the tone for your daughter's relationships with boys and men. The encouragement and support you show her when she's a child will help her become a self-confident, successful woman.

FATHERHOOD

Perhaps the best thing you can do for your children is to take care of yourself and follow the advice in this book. Eat right, exercise, drink only in moderation, and remember that your children are always watching what you do. Besides helping improve the quality and length of your life, you'll be giving your children the tools to do the same.

TIPS TO HELP YOU BE THE KIND OF DAD YOU WANT TO BE
Here are some other tips that can help you be the kind of dad you want to be and that your children need you to be:

- **Jump in!** Don't worry about making a few mistakes. Being a good dad—just like being a good mom—comes with practice. If you really need some help, ask for it, but trust your instincts. Chances are you'll do exactly the right thing.
- **Don't waste a second.** The sooner dads start holding and caring for their babies, the sooner they learn what babies need and what they have to do to comfort them. In the first year, babies mostly need to feel loved. So cuddle, talk, sing, read, and show your baby the sights, sounds, and smells of his or her new world.
- **Be a partner not a helper.** After money, couples argue most about who does what around the house. The more responsibility you take on, the happier your wife will be, the happier you'll be, and the stronger your relationship will be.
- **Stand your ground.** If you're feeling left out, talk to your wife about it. Show her that you're serious about wanting to be an equal participant, and that you're ready and able to do the job.
- **Support breastfeeding.** Ideally, your baby should have nothing but breast milk for the first six months. But nursing is sometimes hard for new moms. Make sure your partner gets plenty of fluids and rest, and encourage her every way you can.
- **Don't forget your relationship.** Before you became parents, you and your wife spent a lot of time together, building your relationship. But now, your baby is the focus of nearly everything you do. Set aside some time every day to talk with your partner—about something other than the baby.

APPENDIX A:
SPECIAL CONCERNS OF AFRICAN-AMERICANS, LATINOS, AND OTHER MINORITIES

Although all men generally live shorter and less-healthy lives than women, African-American men and some other minorities are at even greater risk. African-American men, for example, suffer the worst health of any major population group in the United States, living an average of 6 years less then white men. The reasons for this include lack of health insurance or affordable healthcare, poor education, greater exposure to violence, and genetics.

Because of lack of screening, African-American men are twice as likely to die of prostate cancer as white men.

We've covered many of the racial and ethnic health differences throughout this book, but in this section, we're highlighting issues that are of special concern to men of color.

YOU AND YOUR DOCTOR
African-American and Latino men are less likely than white men to visit a doctor. Again, some of the obstacles include lack of insurance, as well as distrust of the medical establishment. Men's Health Network maintains a list of free and low-cost clinics and information about discounted drugs at: www.healthclinicsonline.com. You can also find information at this site about Medicare, Medicaid, and clinical trials.

DIET AND NUTRITION
Over 60 percent of American men are overweight or obese. Mexican-American men are the most likely to be overweight, followed by white men and African-American men.

EXERCISE AND FITNESS
Despite all these benefits, over half of Americans get less exercise than they should, and a quarter get none at all. African-American and Hispanic men are somewhat less likely to exercise than white men.

SEXUAL HEALTH
African-American men are five times more likely to die of HIV/AIDS than white men. Abstinence is the only sure-fire way to prevent transmission of HIV or other sexually transmitted diseases. However, since abstinence isn't practical for everyone, be sure that you know your partner, always use a latex condom, and avoid drugs or alcohols, which can impair your judgment and increase the chances that you'll engage in unsafe sex.

PROSTATE HEALTH
African-American men are more likely to develop symptoms of benign prostatic hyperplasia (BPH) earlier than white men. They also have the highest rate of prostate cancer in the world—they are at least 50 percent more likely to develop the disease, and twice as likely to die from it, than white men.

APPENDIX A

CARDIOVASCULAR HEALTH
African-American men are about 30 percent more likely than whites to suffer a stroke and 40 percent more likely to die from it.

Among men age 40 to 59, 50 percent of African-Americans and 30 percent of whites have high blood pressure.

African-Americans are less likely to have their cholesterol checked than whites.

Fortunately, African-Americans ages 20 and older are less likely than whites the same age to have high cholesterol. But Mexican-American men are more likely.

DIABETES
Over 18 million Americans have diabetes. Hispanics are much more likely to develop diabetes than whites, and African-Americans are about 60 percent more likely. Asians, Pacific Islanders, and American Indians also have elevated risk.

CANCER
African-American men are more likely to develop cancer than men from any other racial or ethnic group. They also have a far higher death rate from most cancers, including oral and lung cancer.

EMOTIONAL HEALTH AND WELL-BEING
The last few years have seen an increase in the rate of suicide among young African-American males.

ADDICTION AND SUBSTANCE ABUSE
Approximately 27 percent of African-American men smoke, compared to 25 percent of whites.

Among ethnic groups, Hispanics average the most drinks per day, followed by whites, then blacks. African-Americans, however, have the highest alcohol-related death rates of the three groups. African-Americans are also more likely than whites or Hispanics to suffer from alcohol-related liver disease.

Although African-American men are far more likely than whites to use or abuse illegal drugs, the vast majority of men who abuse prescription drugs or OTC drugs are white.

ACCIDENT PREVENTION AND SAFETY
African-American men between the ages of 24 to 40 are much more likely to be murdered than any other ethnic group. The murder rate is 1 in 30 for black men, compared to 1 in 179 for white men. (Compare that with 1 in 132 for black women and 1 in 495 for white women.) Also, men of color are more likely to be employed in manual labor jobs such as construction and other hazardous occupations, so emphasis on workplace safety becomes especially important.

BLOOD DISORDERS: SICKLE CELL ANEMIA
This disease, which affects primarily African-Americans and people of Mediterranean ancestry, is named after the deformed, sickle-shaped red blood

cells it creates. The cells are extremely fragile and break up, causing damage to capillaries (the tiny blood vessels that deliver oxygen throughout the body). That deprives the body's organs and tissues of oxygen.

Symptoms may include headaches, poor circulation, sores on the legs and ankles and stroke. Sickle cell can't be cured, but it can be treated, usually with folic acid, which helps the body produce red blood cells that may replace the damaged cells. Today, most sufferers live past the age of 50.

In order to develop sickle cell, a child must inherit a defective gene from both parents. About 10 percent of African Americans carry one defective gene. That means they won't develop it, but they could pass it on to their children if their spouses are also carriers.

If you are African-American or of Mediterranean descent and planning to start a family, talk to your doctor about getting a blood test to determine whether you carry the gene.

FACIAL HAIR
Beard hair on black men grows curved as does other body hair. After shaving, especially with close shaving, the hair may grow back into the skin, resulting in bumps on the face and neck. Some men find that using an electric razor or not shaving against the grain helps. Those men who suffer from this problem should see a dermatologist for advice.

APPENDIX B: SCREENING AND CHECKUP SCHEDULE

CHECKUPS AND SCREENINGS	WHEN?	AGES 20-39	40-49	50+
PHYSICAL EXAM: Review overall health status, perform a thorough physical exam and discuss health related topics.	Every 3 years Every 2 years Every year	✓	✓	✓
BLOOD PRESSURE: High blood pressure (Hypertension) has no symptoms, but can cause permanent damage to body organs.	Every year	✓	✓	✓
TB SKIN TEST: Should be done on occasion of exposure or suggestive symptoms at direction of physician. Some occupations may require more frequent testing for public health indications.	Every 5 years	✓	✓	✓
BLOOD TESTS & URINALYSIS: Screens for various illnesses and diseases (such as cholesterol, diabetes, kidney or thyroid dysfunction) before symptoms occur.	Every 3 years Every 2 years Every year	✓	✓	✓
EKG: Electrocardiogram screens for heart abnormalities.	Baseline Age 30 Every 4 years Every 3 years		✓	✓
TETANUS BOOSTER: Prevents lockjaw.	Every 10 years	✓	✓	✓
RECTAL EXAM: Screens for hemorrhoids, lower rectal problems, colon and prostate cancer.	Every year	✓	✓	✓
PSA BLOOD TEST: Prostate Specific Antigen is produced by the prostate. Levels rise when there is an abnormality such as an infection, enlargement or cancer. Testing should be done in collaboration with your physician.	Every year		*	✓

CHECKUPS AND SCREENINGS	WHEN?	AGES 20-39	40-49	50+
HEMOCCULT: Screens the stool for microscopic amounts of blood that can be the first indication of polyps or colon cancer.	Every year		✓	✓
COLORECTAL HEALTH: A flexible scope examines the rectum, sigmoid and descending colon for cancer at its earliest and treatable stages. It also detects polyps, which are benign growths that can progress to cancer if not found early.	Every 3-4 years			✓
CHEST X-RAY: Should be considered in smokers over the age of 45. The usefulness of this test on a yearly basis is debatable due to poor cure rates of lung cancer.	Discuss with a physician		✓	✓
SELF-EXAMS: Testicle: To find lumps in their earliest stages. **Skin:** To look for signs of changing moles, freckles, or early skin cancer. **Oral:** To look for signs of cancerous lesions in the mouth. **Breast:** To find abnormal lumps in their earliest stages.	Monthly by self	✓	✓	✓
BONE HEALTH: Bone mineral density test. Testing is best done under the supervision of your physician.	Discuss with a physician			Age 6
TESTOSTERONE SCREENING: Low testosterone symptoms include low sex drive, erectile dysfunction, fatigue and depression. Initial screening for symptoms with a questionnaire followed by a simple blood test.	Discuss with a physician		✓	✓
SEXUALLY TRANSMITTED DISEASES (STDs): Sexually active adults who consider themselves at risk for STDs should be screened for syphilis, chlamydia and other STDs.	Under physician supervision	✓	✓	Discuss

*African-American men and men with a family history of prostate cancer may wish to begin prostate screening at age 40, or earlier.

PLEASE NOTE: Men's Health Network does not provide medical services. Rather, this information is provided to encourage you to begin a knowledgeable dialogue with your physician. Check with your health care provider about your need for specific health screenings.

APPENDIX C: RESOURCES

You can gather more information on these topics from the following sources:

Blueprint for Men's Health
www.blueprintformenshealth.com

Men's Health Network
www.menshealthnetwork.org

Men's Health Month
www.menshealthmonth.org

*Men's Health Week /
National Men's Health Week*
www.menshealthweek.org

Free and/or Low Cost Health Care
www.healthclinicsonline.com

Self Assessment Health Quiz
www.healthselfassessment.com

Men's Health Library
www.menshealthlibrary.org

American Cancer Society (ACS)
www.cancer.org

American Heart Association (AHA)
www.heart.org

American Urological Association (AUA)
www.auanet.org

Women Against Prostate Cancer
www.womenagainstprostatecancer.org

Mr. Dad
www.mrdad.com

*Centers for Disease Control and
Prevention (CDC)*
www.cdc.gov

Gallo Prostate Cancer Center
www.gallocancercenter.com

Male Health Center
www.malehealthcenter.com

National Institutes of Health (NIH)
www.nih.gov

National Cancer Institute (NCI)
www.nci.nih.gov

*National Institute of Mental Health
(NIMH)*
www.nimh.nih.gov

*National Institute of Diabetes and
Digestive and Kidney Diseases (NIDDK)*
www.niddk.nih.gov

Oncology Nursing Society
www.ons.org

Male Breast Cancer Resource Center
www.mensbreastcancer.com